Praise for Ann Douglas's Previous Books

About *The Complete Idiot's Guide® to Canadian His...*

"An irreverent look at our country's past." – Ken McGoogan, *Calgary...*
"Anyone…would benefit from reading it." – Allen Kear, *Winnipeg Free ...*

About *The Unofficial Guide to Having A Baby*:

"Probably the best reference book on the market, giving nonjudgemental and fairly exhaustive information on [a variety of] hot-button topics.… The book lays out as much information as possible and leaves the decision-making to the parents—a surprisingly rare gambit in the bossy world of pregnancy books…"
– Amazon.com Parenting Editor

"…Whether you are looking for the latest information on high tech resources or down-to-earth everyday suggestions, this book has it all. There are money saving tips and charts and checklists to help you through the pregnancy months and get you ready for the delivery, the comments are honest and often touching as Moms talk about disappointments and highs that were part of their experience. A great resource to have on hand." – *Valleykids Parent News*

"Anyone who wants to become a parent may very well be overwhelmed by all the decisions to be made. Fortunately, 'The Unofficial Guide' does a good job of explaining it all. When there is conflicting data (will it be breast or bottle?) the authors present both sides of the argument. There's even a frank discussion about the pros and cons of having a baby, including the truth about the mommy track." – Lisa N. Burby, *Newsday*

About *The Family Tree Detective*:

"A wonderful new book that…takes a child on a fascinating journey of discovery, revealing ways to uncover intriguing pieces of family lore that will delight, entertain, and enlighten young readers." – *Missing Links*

"Every child is bound to discover some stories that are entertaining and rewarding. This can be a summer-long or a life-long enterprise." – Deirdre Baker, *The Toronto Star*

"A wonderful family adventure for any young person…*The Family Tree Detective* makes learning about family ancestry a pleasure." – *Christian Parenting Today*

About *Baby Science*:

"Engagingly educational in focus, *Baby Science*…explains how to guess what babies are trying to say, why their bodies look the way they do, how to hold them and how much they eat and sleep." – *Publisher's Weekly*

"With candid photos and a warm, conversational text, *Baby Science* describes the first extraordinary year of life."– Children's Book of the Month Club

"Douglas helps a youngster navigate Baby World with ease." – Judy W. Winne, *Courier-Post*

"There is plenty to pour over in this brightly illustrated and engaging book." – Susan Perren, *The Globe and Mail*

"*Baby Science* presents the wonderful world of babies…This book would make a great gift for new parents and siblings!" – Karen Jollimore, *Resource Links*

"A useful aid to help siblings adjust to the idea of a newcomer in the house." – Shari Roan, *Los Angeles Times*

"A perfect book for a preschooler with a new sibling, or any young child who is fascinated by babies."
— Cheryl Peterson, *Children's Literature*

"A clearly written, factual book aimed at young children. Peppered with interesting little facts and simple explanations about a baby's first year, it addresses many of the questions kids have about babies."
— *Peterborough Examiner*

About *The Unofficial Guide to Childcare*:

"The childcare bible." — *Chicago Tribune*

"A lot of practical information....This clearly written tome discusses working-parent stress, evaluating out-of-home and in-home childcare options, finding care for a special-needs child, breastfeeding, and part-time care."— *LA Parent*

"*The Unofficial Guide to Childcare* explains how to do a foolproof appraisal of childcare professionals, with plenty of insider secrets and time-saving tips." — *Newsday*

About *Family Finance*:

"Read it before you apply for a mortgage, shop for life insurance, or add to your credit card balance."
— Holly Bennett, Editorial Director, *Today's Parent Group*

"Every parent can profit from reading *Family Finance*...it's an engaging read."
— Helen M. Keeler, *Canadian Living*

About *Sanity Savers*:

"Useful advice and information delivered in a fun, reassuring and practical way." — Laura Bickle, Senior Editor, *Canadian Living*

"When the going gets tough...the tough get tips from Ann Douglas." — Ann Rohmer, Host of City TV's *Breakfast Television*

"An excellent resource for women who are desperate to restore some sanity to their too-busy lives."
— Cheryl Embrett, Senior Editor, *Homemaker's*

"*Sanity Savers* not only helps mothers keep all those balls in the air, but it helps us relax when one inevitably drops." — Louise Brown, Parenting Columnist, *The Toronto Star*

About *The Complete Idiot's Guide® to Canada in the '60s, '70s, and '80s*:

"From mini-skirts to Rubik's Cube, pick up this book and take an entertaining and distinctly Canadian tour of pop culture, politics, and daily life." — Nora Young, host of CBC Radio's *Definitely Not the Opera*

Other Books by Ann Douglas

The Complete Idiot's Guide® to Raising Money-Smart Canadian Kids (Spring 2000)

Sanity Savers: The Canadian Working Woman's Guide to Almost Having It All (1999)

Family Finance: The Essential Guide for Canadian Parents (1999)

The Complete Idiot's Guide® to Canada in the '60s, '70s, and '80s (1999)

The Unofficial Guide to Having A Baby (1999)

The Family Tree Detective: Cracking The Case of Your Family's Story (1999)

The Unofficial Guide to Childcare (1998)

Baby Science: How Babies Really Work (1998)

The Complete Idiot's Guide® to Canadian History (1997)

Coming Soon

Trying Again: A Guide to Pregnancy After Miscarriage, Stillbirth, and Infant Loss (Fall 2000)

The Mother of All Pregnancy Books: The All-Canadian Guide to Conception, Birth, and Everything In Between (Fall 2000)

Before You Were Born: The Inside Story (Fall 2000)

The Incredible Shrinking Woman

Ann Douglas has always been an incredible woman—
and now she's *The Incredible Shrinking Woman*. She's the
girlfriend you can really tell what the number on
that dreaded scale reads, a genuine, voluptuous,
full-figured, work in progress who spent years
studying at the Faculty of Weight Loss of the School
of Hard Knocks. Now she's sensibly working at
reaching her goal weight and sharing her practical
tips and wise insights into what it really takes to
finally graduate into your ideal body. I for one, plan
to join Ann on the rest of her journey. After all,
I have nothing to lose but my hips, thighs, etc, etc, etc.

—Kathy English
Executive Producer, *Lifewise* (www.canoe.ca/lifewise)

The Incredible Shrinking Woman

the Girlfriend's Guide to Losing Weight

Ann Douglas

Prentice
Hall
Canada

A Pearson Company
Toronto

From one incredible shrinking woman to another!

Ann Douglas

Canadian Cataloguing in Publication Data

Douglas, Ann, 1963–

    The incredible shrinking woman: the girlfriend's guide to losing weight

ISBN 0-13-017838-1

1. Weight loss. 2. Reducing diets. I. Title.

RM222.2.D68 2000   613.2'5   C00-930123-2

ISBN 0-13-017838-1

Editorial Director, Trade Division: Andrea Crozier
Acquisitions Editor: Nicole de Montbrun
Copy Editor: Valerie Adams
Production Editor: Jodi Lewchuk
Art Direction: Mary Opper
Cover and Interior Design: Sarah Battersby
Cover Illustrations: Stephanie Powers
Production Manager: Kathrine Pummell
Page Layout: Dave McKay

1 2 3 4 5 WC 04 03 02 01 00

Printed and bound in Canada.

This publication contains the opinions and ideas of its author and is designed to provide useful advice in regard to the subject matter covered. The author and publisher are not engaged in rendering health or other professional services in this publication. This publication is not intended to provide a basis for action in particular circumstances without consideration by a competent professional. The author and publisher expressly disclaim any responsibility for any liability, loss, or risk, personal or otherwise, which is incurred as a consequence, directly or indirectly, of the use and application of any of the contents of this book.

Visit the Prentice Hall Canada Web site! Send us your comments, browse our catalogues, and more. **www.phcanada.com**.

A Pearson Company

To Shari and Krista, for your relentless cheering and unwavering support during my sometimes rocky weight-loss journey. You two are the original "Incredible Shrinking Women" and will always be my heroes.

Contents

Acknowledgments

My name may be the one that's splashed across the front cover of the book (one of the biggest perks of being an author, and something that makes up for all those long days in the lonely writer's garret!), but I'm not the only person who was involved in the making of this book.

First of all, I would like to thank Pamela Steel—chef and cookbook author extraordinaire—for dreaming up such incredible recipes for this book. Pamela, you've proven once and for all that low-fat doesn't have to mean low-taste. A nation full of Incredible Shrinking Women salute you!

I also owe huge calorie-burning hugs to each of the women who agreed to be interviewed during the research of this book: Missy Adams, Ann Baron, Krista Carlson, Dawnette Chadwick, Barb Day, Margaret Diamond, Catherine Donges, Melissa Ellingson, Tammie Falletti, Catherine Garbus, Amy Gist, Kathryn Griffith, Marilyn Hilton, Jenna Jayroe, Bridget Kelley, Heather Lesley, Jill Lindsay, Grace Morrell, Elizabeth Anne Nielsen, Barb Payne, Marti C. Popp, Tammi Raushmier, Susan Reeves, Shari Savage, Amy Swedlo, Susan Therien, and those women who chose to share their experiences anonymously. It's the nitty-gritty tips and heartfelt confessions that you shared with me that bring this book to life. Thank you for sharing your lives and experiences with me so generously.

I also owe a huge debt of thanks to a whole bunch of other people: Robyn Greene and nutritionist Susan Hubay, for their incredibly helpful comments on the manuscript; my editorial assistants Bridget Kelley, Barb Payne, and Janice Kent, for all their behind-the-scenes help (including emergency psychotherapy!); Nicole de Montbrun, Catherine Dorton, Andrea Crozier, and the rest of the wonderful folks at Prentice Hall Canada, for believing in this book enough to acquire it; Valerie Adams, for being gentle with my "baby" during the editing process; Sarah Battersby, for coming up with a fun and eye-catching cover and for working her usual magic on the book's interior; Jodi Lewchuk and Lori McLellan, for overseeing the production process with their usual attention to detail; and—last but not least—those unsung heroes, the sales team, for drumming up so much interest in the book.

Finally, I'd love to thank all those wonderful people in my life who've loved me through thick and through thin. It's your unconditional love and support that finally gave me the courage to shrink.

Ann Douglas
February 2000

Introduction

I had my first encounter with the scale a little over 36 years ago. I weighed in at a positively svelte 5 pounds 13 ounces—the one and only time in my life that I would ever be classified as underweight!

Over the next 35 years, I managed to put on an additional 251 pounds. The pounds didn't show up all at once, of course. They were accumulated gradually over a period of years. Some were packed on during my growing up years, when I was more inclined to hit the couch with a plate of chocolate chip cookies than to ride my bike around the block. Others were gained once I reached adolescence and that hormonal cocktail called puberty made it easier for my body to adorn my butt, hips, and thighs with additional layers of fat cells. And then there was the weight I gained during my first year of university, when I was homesick and miserable. (Let's just say that I majored in muffins.)

Every once in a while I'd go on a fitness kick and do something drastic—like signing up for an aerobics class or treating myself to a pair of high-priced jogging shoes in some mistaken belief that the shoes would make the woman. The aerobics classes were a complete disaster. I was no Jane Fonda. My attempts to keep up with the aerobic instructor's fancy footwork made me feel about as graceful and athletic as an elephant in a tutu. My jogging career was similarly short-lived. I'm a fair-weather exerciser and the Canadian climate gave me a smorgasbord of reasons for hitting the fridge rather than the great outdoors.

By the time I graduated from university, the number on the scale had hit an all-time high of 200 pounds. If you've passed that mark yourself, you know that it's a major milestone: while you can kid yourself into believing that you're "just a little overweight" when the scale reads 199, there's no way you can fool yourself into believing that you're a slightly chubbier version of Pamela Anderson Lee when you weigh in at 200 pounds.

The doctor that I was seeing at the time was a bit of a quack. (Okay, a lot of a quack. He's since lost his medical licence!) He suggested that I start popping cold capsules because they would help to curb my appetite. The caffeine in the capsules left me feeling like a plus-sized version of The Bionic Woman. I was so hyper that I was positively vibrating. Unfortunately, the cold capsule remedy didn't do a thing to help my weight problem. The pounds that I had gained during university seemed to like their new home on my body.

Around this time, my high school sweetheart and I set a date for our wedding. Because my childhood fantasies of walking down the aisle did not include wearing a plus-sized wedding gown, I did what any self-respecting 1980s bride-to-be would have done in my shoes: I went on a diet. I was hungry for an entire summer, chomping on carrot sticks and low-fat fish sticks when what I really wanted was a butter-slathered muffin or a nice, juicy steak. If I caught myself drooling, I'd remind myself that it would all be worth it in the end when I sauntered down the aisle, the perfect picture of bridal beauty.

By some miracle, I managed to drop 25 pounds before the wedding. When I walked down the aisle, I weighed in at a practically Twiggy-like 175 pounds—something that seemed to impress family members to no end. (Weight is a big thing in my family. It's all well and fine to be rich and famous, or to discover a cure for some horrible disease, but what really counts is being skinny. I mean, how many families do you know that work weigh-ins into their family reunions?)

It's a good thing that so many photos were taken of me on my wedding day. They provide permanent proof that I lost weight before I took that momentous stroll down the aisle. Unfortunately, by the time we got the official wedding photos back from the photographer, the bride in the photos didn't look at all like me! The pounds that I had so painstakingly shed during my Summer of Discontent had come back with a vengeance once I started cooking for my brand-new hubby.

Desperate times call for desperate measures. A few months into married life, I decided that it was time for me to get serious about losing weight. I knew that I wanted to start a family in the very near future, and I wasn't too thrilled at the idea of starting out my pregnancy at 200 pounds.

Health was less of a concern for me than good old-fashioned vanity: If those god-awful maternity dresses could make the Demi Moores of the world look frumpy, imagine what they would do to a full-figured gal like me! Little did I know that Demi would ultimately set the bar a few feet higher for image-conscious pregnant women. From the early 1990s onward, we'd be expected to look sexy in the nude!

I managed to get my weight down to 142 pounds—a healthy weight for someone who's 5'6"—but my newfound slimness was short-lived. I got pregnant the very next month! By the time I was wheeled into labour and delivery nine-and-a-half months later, I had managed to gain back every single pound that I had lost before my pregnancy.

I ended up making that trek to labour and delivery four more times over the next decade. Each time I gave birth, I held on to some souvenirs of my pregnancy: a few more stretch marks on my thighs and stomach and a whole lot more pounds on the rest of me.

If I'd stopped gaining weight after each baby was born, I probably would have been able to keep my weight problems under control. Unfortunately, I am one of those chosen few who is able to gain weight rather than lose weight while I'm breastfeeding. For some strange reason, I can't seem to get motivated to exercise during the only 20 minutes a day when I don't have a baby in my arms. To make matters worse, I tend to eat as often as the baby eats—and, as every nursing mother knows—that can mean chowing down on a dozen or more mini-meals each day!

My Disappearing Act

In between babies, I tried to ignore my weight. After all, what was the point of going on a diet if I was about to get pregnant again? (I know. My logic was flawed. Chock it up to years of sleep deprivation!) After I gave birth to my last baby, however, I realized that the moment of truth had finally arrived. It was time to do something about the extra weight that I was carrying around, since I was no longer going to be able to wear my pregnancy "disguise." (Don't know what I'm talking about? Let me explain. Pregnancy makes a great disguise for a large woman. No one can tell if the extra padding on your belly is due to the baby or the quart of Haagen-Daz that you hoovered the night before—or at least that's what I used to tell myself!)

Of course, I didn't make the resolution to lose weight overnight. It actually took me about a year and a half to get serious about making the commitment. I made a few half-hearted efforts to get in shape (like joining a fitness club, but never going!), but then one day something just clicked in my head and I knew that the time had come to lose the extra weight that I had been carrying around for more than 35 years once and for all.

Since that time, I've made some significant lifestyle changes:

- I've started exercising regularly and have discovered to my amazement that "exercise" isn't necessarily a synonym for "torture." (Who knew that weight training and aerobic exercise could actually be fun?)
- I've started paying more attention to what I'm putting in my mouth—monitoring both what types of foods I'm choosing and the amount I'm shovelling in.
- I've put my support team in place—a network of true-blue friends who cheer my weight-loss successes and help me to kick aside the motivational road blocks that seem to crop up from time to time.

- I've spent a lot of time each day focusing on my weight-loss goals—thinking about how much weight I've already lost and looking forward to reaching my goal weight in the very near future.

At some point during the past year, I morphed into The Incredible Shrinking Woman. I stopped thinking of myself as someone who is doomed to be fat forever, but rather as a fit person who is temporarily overweight. That shift in attitude has quite literally changed my life. If I'm having a particularly stressful day and I'm tempted to stuff my face with high-fat foods, I simply take a step back and remind myself that a healthy, normal-weight person would find other ways of dealing with stress than diving into a sea of carbohydrates. Then I pretend to be that person.

That's not to say that I'm living in some sort of weight-loss fantasy world. I still have days when I fall off the wagon and have to force myself to get back on again. What's different now is the fact that I get back on track sooner rather than later. Instead of allowing days, weeks, or months to go by before I get back on my program of healthy living, I force The Incredible Shrinking Woman (the writer formerly known as Ann!) to get her butt back on that wagon right away, like it or not. After all, a naturally slim woman wouldn't allow herself to be seduced by M & Ms for weeks on end, just because she had a fight with her husband. Nor would she hole up in some sleazy-looking coffee shop with a dreamy-looking slice of cheesecake just because her children were giving her grief. If anything, Ms. Slim would lose her appetite momentarily and head to the gym to work off some of the stress. (I know: these naturally slim folks can be a bit hard to stomach at times.)

Why This Book?

The bookstore shelves are overflowing with books that promise to teach you the secrets to losing weight. (The last time I counted, there were more than 700 such titles in print!) So allow me to answer the question that's no doubt running through your head: why does the world need another weight-loss book?

The answer is simple: because this book is different. *The Incredible Shrinking Woman* is the first book that zeroes in on the unique weight-loss challenges faced by women and passes on the types of weight-loss secrets that only your most trusted girlfriends would dare to whisper about. How many guys do you know who would willingly admit to hitting the Tim Horton's drive-thru the night before they started a diet? Or to wearing shorts to the doctor's office on a blustery October day so that the scale would show the lowest possible weight? We're talking about privileged, pink ghetto information here!

Of course, you won't just find out what I've learned from 25 years of studying at the Faculty of Weight Loss of the School of Hard Knocks. You'll also pick up tips and ideas from the dozens of women who agreed to be interviewed for this book—both career dieters and born-again skinnies. You'll find out what they have to say about every conceivable aspect of losing weight—the good, the bad, and the ugly!

Something else that makes this book unique is the fact that it is written by someone who can best be described as a genuine work-in-progress: a voluptuous, full-figured gal who is still in the trenches when it comes to weight loss and who can talk about the joys and challenges of losing weight from that perspective. I haven't forgotten how difficult it can be to stay motivated when the bag of Halloween candy on top of the fridge is calling your name. Nor have I lost sight of the thrill of fitting into the pair of jeans that's been languishing in the back of the closet for as long as you can remember! (Hey, if you hold on to them long enough they come back into style!) I'm still a passenger on this roller coaster ride called weight loss, so I have no choice but to describe the world from the vantage point of a Woman of Size (or is that Thighs?)

What You Won't Find in This Book

What you won't find in this book is a lot of holier-than-thou pontificating. I don't know about you, but I've had it up to here with diet books written by celebrities who were overweight for all of 20 minutes of their adult lives, and who take that as a licence to preach the gospel of slimness to the rest of us!

These folks with their personal trainers and in-home chefs seem to lose sight of the fact that we each have our own personal challenges to deal with when it comes to losing weight. Perhaps you're married to a shift-worker, so you end up eating meals at strange times of the day; you have four kids and find it difficult to get to the gym; and you have a stressful job that requires that you put in an insane number of hours at your desk. (Wait a minute, I just described my own life!) What I'm trying to say is that just as there's no such thing as one-size-fits-all pantyhose—a lesson I learned the hard way a good twenty years ago—there's no such thing as a "one-size-fits-all" weight-loss program. If it was that easy to lose weight, you and I would have done it years ago. Right?

What You Will Find in This Book

What you will find in this book is a smorgasbord of insider information about losing weight—the types of nitty-gritty, no-nonsense advice most books tend to ignore. Rather than feeling like you've committed to reading a 300-page sermon from the latest Oprah-approved weight-loss guru, you'll feel like you're eaves-dropping on a juicy conversation between a bunch of weight-savvy women.

This book will arm you with the facts on

- What it means to be overweight (when there's cause for concern and when there's not).
- What motivates women to lose weight.
- Avoiding fad diets and weight-loss scams that could hurt your body or your budget.
- Designing a food plan and a fitness program that are right for you. (Studies have shown that you're more likely to keep the weight off if you come up with a custom weight-loss program rather than using a ready-made program.)
- Getting your head in the game before you make any lifestyle changes.
- Lining up your own personal cheerleading squad and giving nay-sayers their walking papers.
- Putting your scale in its place.
- Avoiding the motivation zappers that can cause you to fall off the wagon—and picking yourself up if you do happen to fall off.
- What success really means when it comes to weight loss.

You'll also find plenty of useful tools:

- A Body Mass Index table that will help you to set a realistic weight-loss goals.
- A copy of Canada's Food Guide to Healthy Eating.
- A directory of resources that's packed with information of interest to anyone who is serious about losing weight: contact information for dozens of nutri-tion- and fitness-related organizations, web sites, and more.
- A list of recommended readings in case you want to do some further reading on the whole business of losing weight.
- Checklists and tips that are designed to support your weight-loss success.

And you'll come across a few other bells and whistles as you're making your way through the book:

- Practical tips on losing weight, getting active, and leading a healthier lifestyle from "real" women who've been there, done that—and lived to tell!
- The truth about some of the most common myths about dieting and weight loss.

- Pop culture tidbits and trivia that relate to weight loss and dozens of little-known facts about nutrition and fitness.

As you've no doubt gathered by now, this book is unlike any other weight-loss book you've ever read. It's packed with essential tips and tools, and yet it's not afraid to have a little fun along the way. (I think there's some unwritten commandment that states that weight-loss books can't be fun. This won't be the first commandment I've broken, I'm afraid, and it probably won't be the last!)

Ready to morph into an Incredible Shrinking Woman yourself? Grab that measuring tape, hop on that scale, and get ready to hit the next chapter running.

Ann Douglas

1

The Skinny on Being Fat

The latest statistics about U.S. fitness levels are enough to scare you skinny: approximately one in three American women and one in five American men are carrying around enough excess weight to put their health at risk. And as much as we might like to feel superior to the stereotypical "fat American," the situation isn't any better on this side of the border: according to Health Canada, 34 percent of Canadians can be classified as either obese or severely obese.

In this chapter, we're going to talk about why weight is an issue for so many women. Then we'll look beyond the numbers and consider the health implications of being overweight. Next we'll zero in on the top three reasons why women want to lose weight. Then, we'll talk about whether there's such a thing as a good time to lose weight. Finally we'll wrap up the chapter by doing a bit of a reality check and considering what losing weight can—and can't—do for you.

Food for Thought

Wondering who's winning the battle of the bulge? The weight-loss industry, that's who! According to Terri Poulton, author of *No Fat Chicks: How Women Are Brainwashed to Hate Their Bodies and Spend Their Money*, North Americans spend $55 billion per year on weight-loss products and services.

Women and Weight: What's the Problem?

There's no denying it. Women really do have a more difficult time controlling their weight than their male counterparts. So next time some guy you know

Food for Thought

Many seriously overweight individuals are career dieters—people who have tried (and failed) to lose weight time and time again. One recent study revealed that at any given time, one-half of U.S. women and one-third of U.S. men are trying to shed excess pounds.

Food for Thought

Not every culture thinks that the female body's ability to pack on the pounds is necessarily a bad thing. In certain west African countries, girls are housed in special "fattening rooms" where they are encouraged to gain weight in preparation for child-bearing. (This is a far cry from the North American system, where teenage girls are subtly encouraged to diet themselves down to a weight at which their menstrual cycles grind to a halt!)

orders a big slice of cheesecake and then picks at you about your weight, feel free to deck him on behalf of womankind!

So what is it about women and weight gain? Why do so many women find it so easy to put on weight and so difficult to lose it? Do these problems hearken back to that fateful day in the Garden of Eden when Eve was hit with a craving for the forbidden apple? Is weight gain yet another thing we can blame on our blasted hormones? Inquiring minds want to know!

While scientists still haven't put together all of the pieces in the weight-gain puzzle—and they're unlikely to touch the Eve question with a ten-foot pole!—they've certainly identified a number of important factors that help to explain why so many women struggle with their weight more than men do. Here's what they know so far.

(1) Women's Bodies Are Designed to Be Fatter than Men's

While women are blessed with bodies that are capable of performing the ultimate miracle—giving birth to another human being—that functionality doesn't come without a price. Estrogen—the hormone that controls the maturation and the release of an egg each month—is very efficient at laying down fat deposits. This is because a certain amount of fat is required for a woman to maintain her fertility. It doesn't matter if you don't intend to have a baby for another ten or twenty years—or ever, for that matter! Your body is convinced that it's doing you a favour by putting aside enough fat stores to sustain a developing baby through both pregnancy and breastfeeding. And, frankly, if a famine were to hit while you were pregnant or lactating, you'd thank your body for its remarkable foresight.

Fortunately—or unfortunately, depending on how you look at it—famine is the least of our worries here in North America. (According to a recent article in *Life* magazine, the U.S. food industry generates some 3700 calories worth of products a day for every American man, woman, and child, and spends $36 million per year to advertise its products.) Still, even though logic may tell us that famine seems like a fairly remote possibility, our bodies continue to operate in survival mode. Consider what Nancy Etcoff, author of *Survival of the Prettiest: The Science of Beauty*, has to say about our body's inborn survival instincts:

> We are adapted to a world of periodic famines caused by droughts, floods, earthquakes, and the scarcity of plants and game.... That the body has a propensity to store fat, and to respond to food shortages by resetting the metabolism and using food more efficiently, is the bane of dieters but highly adaptive. Or at least it was adaptive before we raised grain-fed animals in penned corrals that yield prime sirloin with 30 percent fat, or refined sugar to create éclairs and doughnuts.

Reproduction also helps to explain why men have leaner bodies than women. Their bodies don't have a vested interest in packing Timbits on to their thighs to ensure some future offspring's survival. (In typical male fashion, they leave that job to the women folk!) What's raging around in men's bodies is testosterone—a hormone that is needed for sperm production and that helps the male body to lay down more muscle tissue.

This is where one of the biggest injustices ever done to womankind comes into play. Since men have more muscle tissue than women and muscle tissue burns more calories than fat, a man can consume more calories in a day than a woman of the same height and weight.

In fact, men are like walking furnaces. While our bodies do whatever they can to store calories as fat, men's bodies try to convert these calories to heat—something which helps to explain one of the greatest mysteries of the modern age: why men and women can never seem to agree about the setting on the electric blanket.

Food for Thought

Wondering how you ended up with those voluptuous, child-bearing hips? Blame it on your hormones. Estrogen redirects fat to certain parts of the female body: the buttocks, the hips, and the thighs. That explains why a typical North American woman is shaped like a pear: size eight on the top but size twelve on the bottom.

Food for Thought

It's not mere coincidence that so many women crave chocolate during the week before menstruation. Some animal researchers believe that foods with high fat and sugar content stimulate the production of endorphins—the natural, opiate-like compounds found in the brain.

The Skinny

Looking for a way to combat those premenstrual munchies? Here are a few tips:

- Take 1200 mg calcium supplements throughout your menstrual cycle. A recent study revealed that women who get adequate amounts of calcium in their diet see a 50% improvement in the severity of their PMS symptoms, including food cravings.

- Turn to complex carbohydrates like whole-grain breads, fruits, and vegetables rather than simple carbohydrates like chips and chocolate bars. Complex carbohydrates will boost your serotonin levels for a couple of hours rather than just making you feel good for a half-hour or so—the downfall of "quick fix" simple carbohydrates.

- Exercise regularly to encourage your body to release plenty of endorphins—the natural, opiate-like substances that can help to improve your mood.

- Avoid caffeine. Not only does caffeine make you more irritable—the last thing you need in the days leading up to your period!—it also tends to increase the severity of PMS symptoms. Studies have shown that women who consume caffeine regularly are four times as likely to suffer from severe PMS as women who don't—so don't be butting in line in front of any grumpy-looking women the next time you're in Tim Horton's!

(2) Women's Bodies Undergo Significant Hormonal Changes Over the Course of a Month

The biological wild card impacts on more than just our bodies' ability to store fat. It also helps to explain why so many women struggle with food cravings during the last week of their menstrual cycle.

Researchers estimate that 80 percent of women experience premenstrual syndrome (PMS) at some point in their lives. One of the most troublesome symptoms of PMS is, of course, food cravings. Many women find that they're able to eat relatively sanely during the first few weeks of their menstrual cycle, but that their usual good eating habits go out the window when the PMS monster arrives on the scene. (Think chocolate!)

A recent study reported in the medical journal *Human Reproduction* explains why we tend to crave truckloads of carbohydrates at this point in our menstrual cycles. Our levels of serotonin—the so-called "feel good" hormone—tend to dip during the week before menstruation kicks in. Since carbohydrates are believed to stimulate the brain to produce serotonin, we crave those types of foods. The only downside to all this premenstrual munching is the fact that it's easy to pack on an extra pound or two each month—weight gain that can really add up to a ten- to twenty-pound weight gain over the course of a year.

(3) Women Tend to Be Less Physically Active than Men

While North Americans as a whole are far less active than they used to be, studies have shown that women are far more likely to be inactive than men: by the time they enter their twenties, just 30 percent of women—as compared to 42 percent of men—are exercising on a regular basis.

You don't have to be a rocket scientist to figure out where the problem lies. Many women are simply too busy to exercise regularly: study after study has shown that working women find themselves struggling with a perpetual time crunch. And then there's the fact that many women have a tendency to put their own needs at the bottom of the list: if something's going to get scratched from the family schedule on a busy Saturday morning, it's more likely to be mom's workout than the kids' hockey games.

Of course, until recently, women didn't have to consciously plan to work exercise into their daily routines. It kind of just happened. It was easy to burn off a couple of thousand calories per day when you were working in the field all day or keeping a house clean without the help of a fleet of labour-saving home appliances. All that has changed in the modern era, notes Claude Bourchard, a Laval University exercise physiologist who was recently interviewed by *Maclean's* magazine: "Mankind's war on muscular effort over the centuries has largely been won. Most of us expend about 300 to 400 fewer calories in energy output each day than we did a half century ago."

> ## The Skinny
>
> "I think one of the biggest keys to taking care of yourself is having time to do so. The only way I can do it is to be up an hour and a half before anyone else so that hopefully when my family responsibilities start, I am exercised, showered, dressed, and have my hair and makeup done. If I'm running behind and looking like hell, I am going to eat badly. That's just the way it is."
>
> — Shari

④ Women Tend to Gain More Weight After Marriage than Men

There's no denying it: that trip to the altar can be bad for your waistline. While men tend to pack on an extra 20 pounds during the first thirteen years of marriage, women tend to gain that and more—a button-popping 25 pounds apiece!

That was certainly Anya's experience. "Married life was good," she recalls. "I loved the creativity of cooking. We both gained 40 pounds that first year."

Kathryn had a similar experience. She also gained weight after she met and married Mr. Right. "I got comfortable," she explains. "I quit exercising and ate what he ate, which was mainly fast food and junk food.

> ## The Skinny
>
> "Although I have always been on the heavy side, my weight really didn't become a problem until after I was married. It was a slow process. I just seemed to gain a little here and there and all of a sudden, here I am 100 pounds overweight."
>
> — Grace

Food for Thought

A recent study by Swedish researchers indicated that 28 percent of women report having an increased interest in sweets during pregnancy. The researchers also found that naturally slim women have less trouble controlling the amount of weight they gain during pregnancy than women with a history of weight problems.

I just assumed I'd stay thin if I didn't pig out too often. Wrong!"

⑤ Pregnancy Is the Greatest Excuse Going for Gaining Weight

Men might find it challenging to keep their weight down if, every couple of years, they were given a licence to pack on an extra 30 pounds. It may sound crazy, but that's exactly what happens to a woman each and every time she becomes pregnant.

Weight gain during pregnancy can be a problem for both veteran dieters and card-carrying skinnies alike. While a lot of the pregnancy weight does disappear once the baby is born, most women find themselves with at least a little "baby fat" to work off. In a perfect world, that extra weight would melt off while you're breastfeeding—after all, wasn't that why you packed the extra weight on to your butt, hips, and thighs in the first place? But, unfortunately, as a recent medical journal article indicated, some women have a tendency to gain weight rather than lose it while they're nursing. Amy, for example, found that she was ravenously hungry, but too tired or busy to fix proper meals. That led to a 20-pound weight gain during her baby's first six months of life.

There are other factors that conspire against you as well when you're in the front lines of new motherhood. As motivated as you may be to lose the extra baby weight, it can be anything but easy to hit the gym when you're trying to meet the demands of a newborn baby. Even if you are blessed with one of those delightful infants who comes programmed to sleep through the night at an early age, you're still going to be more inclined to hit the sack when the baby does rather than grab your runners and head for the gym.

⑥ Women Tend to Gain Weight as They Grow Older

Depressed with all this talk about weight gain during pregnancy? We haven't even got to the good stuff yet: aging!

Believe it or not, aging is at the root of the weight problems of a large number of older women. Here's why. From age 30 onward, reduced activity levels and hormonal changes cause us to lose lean muscle mass at the rate of about half a pound per year. This causes our metabolic rate to slow down, meaning that we burn off calories less efficiently. Unless we clue in to what's happening and reduce our caloric indicate appropriately—or, even better, exercise regularly so that we can maintain as much lean muscle mass as possible—the pounds can creep on unexpectedly.

To make matters worse, we're hit with a rather nasty curve ball as the years march on. The hormonal changes of menopause tend to cause a shift in fat deposits from hip to belly, something that causes middle-aged women to look less like pears and more like apples. Not only does this make it more difficult to find comfortable jeans, it's also not good for your health. Studies have shown that women who have apple-shaped bodies are at greater risk of health problems like heart disease, high blood pressure, diabetes, and certain types of cancers than women with pear-shaped bodies. (See the detailed discussion on the health consequences of being overweight later in this chapter.) That's why most doctors agree that a woman whose waist measures more than 35 inches needs to think seriously about getting rid of the extra weight she is carrying around.

More Bad News

Of course, not all of women's weight woes can be blamed on the mere fact of being female. A lot of our weight problems are more the result of our eating habits than the fact that we are carrying around two X chromosomes.

Don't understand what I'm talking about? Let me explain. Even though the grocery stores shelves are overflowing with low-calorie, low-fat foods, the North American love affair with high-calorie, high-fat foods continues. Consider the evidence for yourself:

- According to the Canadian Restaurant and Foodservices Association, french fries were the most-ordered item in Canadian restaurants in 1998 for the second year running. The top ten list was also padded with plenty of other high-fat choices: croissants, hamburgers, pizza, cheesecake, donuts, and ice cream. (See Table 1.1.)

TABLE 1.1

THE TEN MOST ORDERED RESTAURANT ITEMS IN CANADA IN 1998

1. French fries	6. Sandwiches
2. Unsweetened baked goods	7. Desserts
3. Hamburgers	8. Sweetened baked goods
4. Salads	9. Oriental stir-fry
5. Pizza	10. Ice cream and frozen yogurt

Source: *The Globe and Mail.*

• Most of us have long-since forgotten what a "normal" serving size is. Bucket-sized containers of soda pop, super-sized chocolate bars, and gigantic restaurant entrées are fast becoming the norm. One convenience store chain in the U.S. has actually introduced a 2.5 litre drink of soda pop that is appropriately named "the Beast." (The biggest thing we can find north of the border, on the other hand, is the comparatively minuscule 1.9 litre "Double Gulp.") At the same time, the standard restaurant plate has grown from 10 inches to 12 inches to accommodate increasingly larger serving sizes. (No wonder! If you plunked your 12 ounce steak on the smaller-sized plate, you'd hardly have room for the baked potato, onion rings, curly fries, dinner roll, and cob of corn—those delicious fat-slathered side-dishes that can easily triple the calorie count of your family-sized serving of steak!)

Clearly, it's time for both restaurant plates and fast-food serving containers to go on a diet. But with convenience stores, fast-food restaurants, and even fine dining establishments seemingly convinced that "more is better," it could be a very long time before a "small"-sized serving of soda pop is anything but huge!

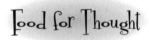

Not everyone who thinks she is overweight actually needs to lose weight. A study conducted by researchers at the Melpomene Institute in the U.S. revealed that 97 percent of women who considered themselves to be slightly overweight were actually within the normal weight range for their height.

How Fat Is Too Fat?

The man in your life tells you that he likes your curves and your best friend insists you really don't need to lose much weight at all. If you can't get the truth from those nearest and dearest to you, how do you go about deciding whether or not you actually need to lose weight?

Fitness experts typically rely on one of two tools when deciding whether or not a particular person would benefit from dropping a few pounds: (1) the Body Mass Index (BMI) and (2) body fat measurements.

Body Mass Index (BMI)

There's no denying it: the BMI is a vast improvement over its predecessor, the insurance company height-weight table. For one thing, it's more realistic: it tends to give people a little more leeway when determining what their "ideal weight" should be. For another, it tends to be a lot less confusing to use.

You see, the old height-weight charts used to provide weight ranges for people with small, medium, and large frames. The problem was that most people couldn't figure out what their frame size actually was, so they didn't know which set of weight ranges they should be aiming for. (I, of course, used the choice of three frames to my advantage. If I was allowed to weigh a good twenty to thirty pounds more if I had a large frame, then big-boned I would be! It seemed a small price to pay in order to be allowed to carry a few extra pounds without the usual guilt.)

Still, despite the fact that you could buy yourself a few extra pounds by fudging your frame size a little, the pre-BMI days were definitely not the good old days for full-figured gals like me. Today I can pull out my handy-dandy BMI table and see that a healthy weight for someone my height—5'6"—can fall anywhere between 124 and 148 pounds. While the odds of me ever weighing in at 124 pounds again are virtually nil (for Pete's sake, I haven't weighed that little since I was in the seventh grade!), 148 pounds seems like a perfectly achievable goal. It's just a few pounds heavier than I was during that magical six-week period in my pre-childbearing life when I was at a healthy weight. (It's also a whole lot more realistic than the virtually unattainable maximum weight of 128 pounds that the old height-weight tables wanted me to achieve.)

So now that we've agreed upon the fact that the BMI is a good thing—or at least a much better thing than anything else that has come before—let's talk about what it means and how it is calculated.

Basically, the BMI is a number that relates your weight to your height. The basic formula works like this:

$$\text{BMI} = \text{weight (kg)} \div \text{height (centimetres)}^2$$

If you're still resisting the metric conversion and continuing to weigh yourself in pounds, use this formula instead: $155 \times 64^2 \times 704.5$

$$\text{BMI} = \text{weight (pounds)} \div \text{height (inches)}^2 \times 704.5$$

If you're a math junkie, you can have some fun crunching these numbers for yourself; if you're not, don't sweat it. I've done the work for you. (See Table 1.2.)

Now let's stop and consider what these numbers actually mean:

- A BMI that's between 20 and 25 is considered to be ideal from a health standpoint. If your BMI falls within this range, take this book back to the bookstore right now. You don't need it! (My publisher hates it when I say

TABLE 1.2

BODY MASS INDEX

Height (Inches)	19	20	21	22	23	24	25	26	27	28	29	30	31	32	33	34
			HEALTHY WEIGHT					OVERWEIGHT WARNING ZONE		OVERWEIGHT HEALTH RISK				OBESE		
	Body Weight (pounds)															
58	91	96	100	105	110	115	119	124	129	134	138	143	148	153	158	162
59	94	99	104	109	114	119	124	128	133	138	143	148	153	158	163	168
60	97	102	107	112	118	123	128	133	138	143	148	153	158	163	168	174
61	100	106	111	116	122	127	132	137	143	148	153	158	164	169	174	180
62	104	109	115	120	126	131	136	142	147	153	158	164	169	175	180	186
63	107	113	118	124	130	135	141	146	152	158	163	169	175	180	186	191
64	110	116	122	128	134	140	145	151	157	163	169	174	180	186	192	197
65	114	120	126	132	138	144	150	156	162	168	174	180	186	192	198	204
66	118	124	130	136	142	148	155	161	167	173	179	186	192	198	204	210
67	121	127	134	140	146	153	159	166	172	178	185	191	198	204	211	217
68	125	131	138	144	151	158	164	171	177	184	190	197	203	210	216	223
69	128	135	142	149	155	162	169	176	182	189	196	203	211	216	223	230
70	132	139	146	153	160	167	174	181	188	195	202	209	216	222	229	236
71	136	143	150	157	165	172	179	186	193	200	208	215	222	229	236	243
72	140	147	154	162	169	177	184	191	199	206	213	221	228	235	242	250
73	144	151	159	166	174	182	189	197	204	212	219	227	235	242	250	257
74	148	155	163	171	179	186	194	202	210	218	225	233	241	249	256	264
75	152	160	168	176	184	192	200	208	216	224	232	240	248	256	264	272
76	156	164	172	180	189	197	205	213	221	230	238	246	254	263	271	279

things like that.) And if your BMI is below 20, you are underweight and should probably consider trying to put on a few pounds.

• A BMI of between 25 and 29.9 may indicate that you're overweight and consequently at increased risk of developing certain types of health problems including cardiovascular disease and diabetes. (You'll notice that I said, "may." That's because the BMI formula isn't smart enough to figure out how much of your weight is due to muscle mass as opposed to fat. If you're a highly fit person — perhaps someone with a BMI between 25 and 27 — you may end up showing up as "overweight" on the BMI table when you're actually a living and breathing advertisement for good health. This is one of those situations in which the numbers can and do lie.)

35	36	37	38	39	40	41	42	43	44	45	46	47	48	49	50	51	52
167	172	177	181	186	191	196	201	205	210	215	220	224	229	234	239	244	248
173	178	183	188	193	198	203	208	212	217	222	227	232	237	242	247	252	257
179	184	189	194	199	204	209	215	220	225	230	235	240	245	250	255	261	266
185	190	195	201	206	211	217	222	227	232	238	243	248	254	259	264	269	275
191	196	202	207	213	218	224	229	235	240	246	251	256	262	267	273	278	284
197	203	208	214	220	225	231	237	242	248	254	259	265	270	278	282	287	293
204	209	215	221	227	232	238	244	250	256	262	267	273	279	285	291	296	302
210	216	222	228	234	240	246	252	258	264	270	276	282	288	294	300	306	312
216	223	229	235	241	247	253	260	266	272	278	284	291	297	303	309	315	322
223	230	236	242	249	255	261	268	274	280	287	293	299	306	312	319	325	331
230	236	243	249	256	262	269	276	282	289	295	302	308	315	322	328	335	341
236	243	250	257	263	270	277	284	291	297	304	311	318	324	331	338	345	351
243	250	257	264	271	278	285	292	299	306	313	320	327	334	341	348	355	362
250	257	265	272	279	286	293	301	308	315	322	329	338	343	351	358	365	372
258	265	272	279	287	294	302	309	316	324	331	338	346	353	361	368	375	383
265	272	280	288	295	302	310	318	325	333	340	348	355	363	371	378	386	393
272	280	287	295	303	311	319	326	334	342	350	358	365	373	381	389	396	404
279	287	295	303	311	319	327	335	343	351	359	367	375	383	391	399	407	415
287	295	304	312	320	328	336	344	353	361	369	377	385	394	402	410	418	426

- A BMI of 30 or more indicates that you're obese and consequently are at even higher risk of experiencing of health problems as a result of your weight.

Of course, not everyone agrees that 25 should be the cutoff mark between what's considered "healthy" and what's deemed "possibly overweight." Even the former U.S. Surgeon General C. Everett Koop makes a rather convincing case for giving would-be dieters a bit of breathing room by pumping the magic number up to 27. (That would allow me to weigh in at as much as 167 pounds—a weight that I actually do feel very good at—rather than dieting down to a svelte-for-me 142 pounds.)

Food for Thought

Wondering how your BMI measures up to that of other Canadians? A Health Canada study conducted in 1994 and 1995 revealed that while 43% of Canadians are at a healthy weight (i.e., their BMIs fall between 20 and 24.9) and 8% are actually underweight (their BMIs are less than 20), 30% of Canadians are considered to be overweight (BMIs of 27 or more) and another 19% of Canadians may be overweight, too (with BMIs between 25 and 27). Here's another interesting fact to chew on, courtesy of the folks at Health Canada: while women are far more likely to worry about their weight than men are, only 26% of women (as opposed to 35% of men) were actually overweight.

Body Fat Measurements

You've no doubt heard about the lengths that some people go to in order to obtain precise body fat measurements: they submerge themselves in special dunk tanks that are designed for this purpose or they allow someone to pass electrical currents through their bodies!

"So what's wrong with the old bathroom scale?" you're probably wondering. For one thing, bathroom scales are notoriously inaccurate. My old one weighed about seven pounds heavier than the scale at the gym, while my new one consistently puts me about five pounds lighter. (You can see why the first scale got the old heave-ho while the new one has earned a place of honour in my kitchen!)

But even if the number on the bathroom scale—or the number on the scale at the gym, for that matter—is accurate, it really doesn't tell you how fat you are. You see, all that number (and consequently your BMI) is telling you is how much your bones, blood, fat, muscle tissue, and so on weigh. What you want to know is how much of your body is composed of fat.

If you decide to go the body fat measurement route, you can expect to undergo one or more of the following three tests:

- Underwater weighing (you are lowered into a tank of water on a chair attached to a scale)
- Skinfold measuring (calipers are used to measure the thickness of your skin at certain points on your body, typically in your upper arm, under your shoulder blade, just above the hip, at the waist, and on the thighs)
- Bioelectrical or electrical impedance (electrodes are placed on your hands and feet and an electric current is sent through your body)

The Skinny

Don't take your body fat measure as the gospel truth if you happen to have the test performed during the four to six days before your period. Women typically experience a two- to five-pound water-weight gain just before their periods, something that can throw that body fat measurement out by as much as 3 mm.

Unfortunately, none of these three tests is perfect:

- Underwater weighing can be prohibitively expensive and it's definitely a no-no for anyone who's claustrophobic or who has a fear of water.
- Skinfold measuring is only as accurate as the person performing the test. What's more, it isn't a good choice for anyone over the age of 55 (the point in life when your subcutaneous fat—the fat right under your skin—begins to thin, making these types of measurements inaccurate).
- Bioelectrical or electrical impedance is less than reliable, even though it sounds wonderfully high-tech and impressive. Besides, not everyone is eager to line up for the opportunity to have an electrical current passed through their body— even though the test is apparently painless and perfectly safe.

While BMI figures and body fat measurements can provide you with a general idea of your overall fitness level, what they can't tell you is whether your health will improve if you lose a certain amount of weight. Only your doctor can tell you that, based on his or her specific knowledge of your medical history and your current lifestyle. If, for example, you are experiencing such weight-related problems as cardiovascular disease, type two diabetes, osteoarthritis, gallstones, stress incontinence, or polycystic ovarian syndrome (a gynecological condition that can wreak havoc on your attempts to become pregnant), your doctor may recommend that you make a concerted effort to lose weight. If, however, you're just a few pounds overweight and you're in otherwise excellent health, your doctor may not think it's necessary for you to make any radical lifestyle changes—yet another good reason for checking in with your doctor before you embark on a new fitness program.

The Skinny

Don't put away all those measuring devices away yet. There's one more measure that doctors like to do when assessing the health risks posed by the amount of weight someone is carrying. Since people whose fat is concentrated primarily in the abdominal area (the so-called "apples" of the world) are believed to be at greater risk of developing certain types of health problems than those folks who carry their extra weight on their hips, thighs, and buttocks (the so-called "pears" of the world), doctors take into account an individual's hip-to-waist ratio. You can figure out your hip-to-waist ratio for yourself by grabbing a tape measure and measuring your waist at its narrowest point and your hips at their widest point. Women with waist-to-hip ratios of more than 0.8 or men with waist-to-hip ratios of more than 1.0 are considered to be "apples," who are at higher-than-average risk of developing weight-related health problems.

The Magic Number

The experts say that it doesn't make sense to get too fixated on a particular goal weight when you're just embarking on a weight-loss program. (This is especially true for people who've got a lot of weight to lose and who may become discouraged if their target weight seems to be too far away from their present weight.) They recommend instead that people focus on a more immediate goal—like dropping ten pounds, for example.

While this strategy works for some people, others really like to have a magic number in their head that tells them how much weight they're going to lose. I have to confess that I've been focusing on reaching 142 pounds since the moment I started my weight-loss program. In fact, I made photocopies of an old photo of myself at 142 pounds—the only one I could find shows me holding a bunch of zucchinis!—and hung them around the house. There's one on the side of the fridge, one on the wall above my desk, and one on the bookshelves in my study. My husband and kids thought it was a pretty weird thing for me to do, especially figuring how prominently the zucchinis figure in the photo, but it's certainly worked for me. If I'm ever tempted to have a late-night fling with some fly-by-night high-fat food lurking in my refrigerator, that photo of the younger-and-slimmer me usually makes me think twice before I open my mouth.

If you feel like you need to have some magic number designated as your goal weight—and, frankly, some women do prefer to focus on long-term rather than short-term goals—you might want to choose as your goal weight the lowest weight that you've been able to maintain during your adult life for a year or more without struggling.

As much as you might like to reach new levels of slenderness, it doesn't make a lot of sense to pick a weight that is so low that you'll have trouble maintaining it. That's just setting yourself up for frustration and failure—the last thing you need! Amy, a life-long dieter, learned this the hard way after losing a lot of weight during her university years: "I dieted and exercised until I managed to get that 28-inch waist I had been dying to have. But I couldn't eat anything that was remotely interesting or fun without instantly gaining weight. That was not success because it wasn't comfortable."

The Three Big Reasons Why Women Want to Lose Weight

Looking for some reasons to get serious about losing weight this time around? Here are the three biggest reasons why most women want to lose weight.

(1) To Be Healthier

Health considerations are the number-one weight-loss motivation for women who have a significant amount of weight to lose. (For women who have just a few pounds to lose, the key consideration tends to be appearance rather than health.)

Melissa was motivated to lose weight out of concern about the impact that her weight might have on her fertility. She's hoping to start a family soon, but she knows that seriously overweight women tend to have more difficulty conceiving than normal-weight women.

Shari decided to get serious about losing weight this year because she was worried about the health implications of being significantly above her ideal weight: "Being 43 makes me realize I don't exactly have forever to take care of the problem. And I want to still be young enough to enjoy having a fit body when I get one."

Melissa and Shari are wise to make health one of their key motivations for losing weight. Some studies have indicated that women who are motivated by health rather than appearance are more likely to stick to their weight-loss programs than women who try to lose weight for other reasons. Here are four great benefits to losing weight "for the health of it."

You Can Reduce Your Risk of Heart Disease

Cardiovascular disease is the number one cause of premature death in Canada, resulting in some 79 000 deaths each year. Obesity is responsible for a significant number of these deaths: according to one U.S. study, people who are seriously overweight have a 75% greater chance of experiencing a stroke than people who are at a normal weight.

There are a number of reasons that explain why overweight people are at increased risk of developing cardiovascular problems. (Nearly 70 percent of people who are diagnosed with heart disease are overweight.)

- Overweight people are more likely to have high blood pressure—a major risk factor for both heart disease and stroke—than people who are at a healthy weight.

> **The Skinny**
>
> "My major motivation for getting healthy is my daughters: they are six and five. I want them to understand how important it is to be healthy. I never want them to go through this struggle."
> — Tammie

> **Food for Thought**
>
> According to Health Canada, obesity is responsible for one in five deaths in Canada.

- They may have higher-than-average levels of cholesterol and triglycerides (blood fats), something that can result in buildups in the coronary arteries (the arteries leading to the heart). The arteries narrow as a result of this buildup of gunk, something that prevents the heart muscle from getting the oxygen and nutrients it needs to operate properly. A heart attack occurs when the arteries become so constricted that they finally close off, or a blood clot that would normally pass through an unobstructed artery gets stuck somewhere along the way.
- They are at higher-than-average risk of becoming diabetic—a condition that increases your chances of developing heart disease.

Don't make the mistake of assuming that cardiovascular disease is just a guy thing, by the way. In the U.S., it's thought to be responsible for 42 percent of women's deaths, as compared to 32 percent of men's deaths.

You Can Reduce Your Chances of Developing Diabetes

If you've got a family history of diabetes and you're significantly overweight, you owe it to yourself to get rid of some of the extra pounds. Failing to do so is like waving a red flag in front of a bull—but in this case, the bull is a disease can cause premature death, heart disease, kidney disease, stroke, and blindness.

The statistics speak for themselves:

- Nearly 80 percent of people who develop type two diabetes are obese.
- Overweight people are twice as likely to develop diabetes as normal-weight people.
- Eleven percent of Canadians over the age of 65 are diabetic.
- Diabetes is responsible for more than 5000 deaths in Canada each year.

It's not hard to figure out why diabetes can do so much damage to the body. Insulin—the substance that diabetics have trouble producing—plays a key role in regulating blood sugar levels and storing fat. It actually functions as an after-dinner maid service, clearing blood sugar and fat byproducts out of the bloodstream. If you don't produce adequate quantities of top-quality insulin, you're left with a lot of gunk floating around in your blood. Over time, this can cause significant damage to your body's internal organs.

Food for Thought

Scientists estimate that between 30% and 40% of cancers could be eliminated if people exercised regularly, ate properly, and maintained a healthy weight.

You Can Cut Your Chances of Getting Cancer

Overweight women are at increased risk of developing uterine, gallbladder, cervical, ovarian, breast, and colon cancer. They are also at increased risk of dying from certain types of cancers as compared to normal-weight women.

You Can Reduce Your Risk of Developing Other Types of Health Problems

A whole smorgasbord of ailments can be blamed on obesity. By losing even just part of the extra weight you're carrying, you can reduce your chances of developing the following types of health problems:

- **High blood pressure (a.k.a. "hypertension").** Being obese more than doubles your chances of developing high blood pressure.
- **Respiratory problems.** Being obese puts you at increased risk of developing respiratory problems.
- **Gout (painful joint problems caused by excess uric acid).** Obesity makes it harder for your body to excrete uric acid, something that can lead to gout.
- **Osteoarthritis (wearing away of the cartilage that cushions the joints).** The pressure of carrying around extra weight can cause symptoms ranging from mild stiffness and aching joints to severe pain and disability.
- **Gallstones.** Women who are more than 40 percent over their ideal weight are one-third more likely to develop gallstones than normal-weight women of the same age.
- **Sleep apnea (interrupted breathing during sleep).** Overweight people are more likely to experience sleep apnea—a condition that can cause everything from daytime sleepiness to snoring at night to heart failure! (The problem is caused by excess fat tissue around the neck that closes off the airway, causing breathing problems while you are sleeping.)
- **Decreased fertility.** Overweight women tend to have more difficulty conceiving than normal-weight women. A study at the University of South Carolina at Charleston revealed that 76 percent of overweight women with fertility problems managed to conceive when they reached their ideal weights.
- **Psychological problems.** Overweight people are at increased risk of experiencing such psychological problems as depression, isolation, and low self-esteem. (Of course, this is due in large measure to the "fat prejudice" that many overweight women face on a day-to-day basis.)

The Skinny

Eager to avoid the agony of gallstones? (And, frankly, who could blame you?) Welcome to the weight-loss world's version of a Catch 22. You're at increased risk of developing them if you're overweight, but losing weight too quickly can also cause them to become a problem for you. So what's a health-conscious gal to do? Lose weight slowly, the experts say. You're less likely to develop gallstones if you aim for a weight loss of about a pound a week than if you go on a crash diet.

The Skinny

Don't be surprised if your reasons for wanting to lose weight change over time. While she started out wanting to lose weight for health reasons, Dawnette's focus has changed now that she's getting closer to her goal: "These days, my key motivation is to fit my clothes and look better. Before it was because the weight was so hard on my knees and back."

② To Look Good

This one's a real no-brainer: another big reason why many women want to lose weight is to look better.

While health is Bridget's main reason for wanting to lose weight, she's also motivated by a desire to improve her physical appearance. "I would dearly love to look good, too: younger, sexier, to be able to wear whatever I saw that I liked—even a miniskirt for once!" she confesses. "I am feeling very 'middle-aged' right now: frumpy, tired, nondescript. I hate that!"

Marilyn is also hoping to be able to change what she sees in the mirror: "I've reached the point where I'm thoroughly disgusted with myself. None of my clothes fit, I look and feel 'matronly,' my husband doesn't answer me when I ask him if I look fat, and I feel like I've had a reverse liposuction."

Melissa wants to be able to dress more stylishly: "I want to be able to get into smaller clothes and have some cute outfits that don't cost $100 from the 'fat lady's store.'"

It's not hard to figure out why "looking good" is such a powerful motivation for so many women. For the past few decades, it's been open season on fat people. Journalist Natalie Angier described the problem in a recent article in the *New York Times*: "People who would never publicly confess to racism have no qualms about expressing revulsion for the obese."

Of course, it's not just the Joan Riverses of the world who like to have fun at the expense of fat people—although Joan did take the "art" of the fat joke to previously unimagined heights. The tabloids have had great fun—and made huge amounts of money—at Oprah and Elizabeth Taylor's expense. (Think it's hard to gain 20 pounds and have family members and friends notice? Imagine what it must be like to find your picture slapped on the front page of the *National Enquirer* for committing the

Food for Thought

According to Terri Poulton, author of *No Fat Chicks: How Women Are Brainwashed to Hate Their Bodies and Spend Their Money*, women's clothing stores routinely carried garments up to size 18, and sometimes even size 20, up until the 1960s. Then the Twiggy phenomenon hit North America and women were expected to have slender, boyish figures. By the 1990s, the largest size carried by many women's clothing stores was a size 14.

"crime" of gaining weight!) And while we Canadians like to pretend that we're above all that American fat-bashing nastiness, we don't mind snickering a little when some of our country's best-known comedians choose to poke fun at plus-sized Maritime songstress Rita MacNeil.

The fact is that it's become downright respectable to poke fun at fat people—and it's only going to get worse! I recently heard a radio interview in which a group of health promoters were talking about ways to get the weight message across to an increasingly overweight society. The group agreed that soft-sell messages weren't working: that it was time to pull out the big guns and start shaming overweight people into losing weight! Can't you just see how this could be played out in the fast food drive-thru? You'd place your order for a burger and large fries and then a booming Big Brother-type voice from inside the restaurant would announce, "I don't think so, Miss Piggy! You're getting a large garden salad and a Diet Coke. Now drive ahead."

What many people don't seem to realize is that fat discrimination can do a number on your entire life— not just your ego. (Just to clarify: I'm not just talking about the fallout from schoolyard bullying that happened years ago—although many overweight people have that to deal with as well: I'm talking about the day-to-day abuse that many overweight adults experience each and every day of their lives.) Consider what the latest research has to say about fat discrimination in North America.

Food for Thought

There certainly seems to be a double standard when it comes to the battle of the bulge. Society is far more willing to cut men a bit of slack in the weight department than they're willing to cut women. While the media seems willing to excuse U.S. President Bill Clinton—the so-called "First Jogger"—for allowing his weight to creep up a little from time to time, it didn't choose to extend the same courtesy to Kim Campbell, the first female Prime Minister of Canada. Instead, according to Terry Poulton, author of *No Fat Chicks: How Women Are Brainwashed to Hate Their Bodies and Spend Their Money,* the media lampooned Campbell for what was at most "moderate pudginess."

- A study at the Harvard School of Public Health found that obese women were 20% less likely to marry and 10% more likely to be living in poverty than their slimmer counterparts.
- A study conducted by University of Pittsburgh psychology professor Irene Frieze concluded that grossly overweight females are penalized more heavily on the job than grossly overweight males.

- According to Terri Poulton, author of *No Fat Chicks: How Women Are Brainwashed to Hate Their Bodies and Spend Their Money*, 60% of overweight North American women report that they've been denied employment because of their weight, and one-third report that they've been passed over for promotions and raises.

So "looking good" isn't just about fitting into a dress of a particular size (although, frankly, that's kind of a nice perk!), it's also about having power in our society—power that fat women crave.

③ Because They're Sick of Being Fat

Some women decide to lose weight because they're simply sick of being fat.

That was certainly the case for Kathryn, who has dropped 70 pounds over the past year: "I didn't feel comfortable with myself at 212 pounds," she recalls. "I kept feeling like there was a thin person inside me and I had to find that person and bring her out." Kathryn became motivated to set that thin person free after what can best be described as the beach vacation from hell! At that point, she was at her all-time high of 212 pounds—a weight that left her feeling like "Orca the whale" next to her short, thin sisters-in-law. She felt so fat and ugly that she decided to start her weight-loss program the day after she got home. She's never looked back.

Jenna—who has lost 90 pounds over the past year—decided to make some changes to her life after realizing that she was sitting on the sidelines more and more because of her weight: "My motivation was a convention that many of my friends attended. I really wanted to go, but I was too ashamed of my size to consider it. At that point, something in me clicked. I said to myself, 'That's it. I will never miss another thing because I'm too fat.'"

Tammie's motivation for starting her own weight-loss program was similar to Jenna's: "I want to run in the park, swing in the swings, ride rides at amusement parks, and not worry about whether restaurants have booths that I can fit into. I want to be able to go anywhere without any worries."

Heather—who is currently carrying around about 70 extra pounds—is equally determined to lose weight

The Skinny

"My motivation this time is to break free of the chains that obesity has placed on me. Whether these chains are physical—because I just can't do things I like—or emotional—because of fear of what others will say or of hurting myself—or social—because being fat limits opportunity, there are still things in life that I want to do that I am not doing. My motivation is to live life to the fullest and to stop apologizing for who I am."

— Catherine

this time: "I have a million motivations to lose weight. I always have. This time it's even more urgent: I am at a weight I never imagined I'd see in my worst nightmares. I can't begin to describe the mortification I feel every minute of every day at being this weight. My weight problem has affected ever single facet of my life and I've hit rock bottom."

Is This the "Perfect Time" to Lose Weight?

Are you waiting for "the perfect time" to come along so that you can finally do something about your weight? If you are, I've got news for you, sister. There's no such thing as the perfect time! No matter how much you'd like to be able to start your weight-loss program during a completely stress-free time in your life—a time when you've got no money worries, you and your partner are getting along just swimmingly, and your boss is showering you with praise!—it's unlikely that all of your problems are going to clear the deck long enough for you to shed the extra pounds.

Consider what Jill, a veteran dieter, has to say about the wisdom of waiting for "the perfect time" to lose weight: "To postpone this effort only adds more pounds to the caboose. I used to start diets on Mondays or the first of the month. Or I'd wait for a stressful event to be over: a move, a wedding, a holiday. Now I realize that that's foolish: there will always be birthdays and holidays in life. Thin people enjoy them without gorging themselves. So can I!"

That said, you do need to be in the right frame of mind in order to lose weight successfully—and it's hard to be in that frame of mind if you're in the middle of a crisis at work or a messy divorce. "Personal readiness is the key," explains Jenna. "If there is something happening in your life that occupies your thoughts, it's going to be difficult to focus on weight loss. Although we can make small changes that don't disrupt our lives, a serious focus on losing weight requires a great deal of concentration, time, and effort."

Kathryn agrees that your head has to be in the game if you're really serious about losing weight. For her, what was critical was self-acceptance: "I believe that you must reach a certain peace with yourself to be ready to go on a weight-loss program. Losing weight is an entirely personal choice. This choice cannot be made because someone else wants you to or because

The Skinny

"The right time to lose weight is when we love ourselves enough to do what is right for our bodies."

— Krista

The Skinny

"The right time to lose weight is when you really believe you have to make a change, when you are not happy with yourself and can't live that way one more day."

— Catherine

you feel you have to because of outside influences. It has to be for you and only you. I started losing weight because I wanted to get back in touch with the me I always imagined I could be. Sure, that's partly cosmetic—wanting to look more attractive—but it's also about feeling good about myself. And after losing 70 pounds, I am more confident. I feel like a strong, centred woman. Now that I've lost this weight, I feel like I can do anything."

Great Expectations: What Losing Weight Can and Can't Do for You

It's easy to go a little crazy when you're fantasizing about how losing weight is going to change your life: to convince yourself that every aspect of your life will dramatically improve the moment the "right" number shows up on the scale.

You know how the weight-loss fantasy game works. You paint an outlandish picture of what life will be like on that wonderful day when you finally reach your goal weight. (If you're really good at this, your fantasy also includes a good dose of revenge for all those people who've hassled you about your weight over the years.)

Here's a typical fantasy. You're going to look drop-dead gorgeous—so drop-dead gorgeous that complete strangers will stop you on the street to ask how you're related to Cindy Crawford. Your boss will decide that your talents on the job have been grossly undervalued all these years and will give you a nice juicy raise and an even better promotion. The man in your life will suddenly realize how guilty he's been of taking you for granted and will whisper those three little words that every woman loves to hear: "I was wrong." And—now here's the real icing on the cake!—all those naturally skinny people who've been bugging you about your weight all these years will suddenly discover to their horror that they've developed pot bellies of their own!

As delicious as these weight-loss fantasies can be to savour during those hair-raising moments when there's nothing standing between you and a mouth-watering slice of chocolate chip cookie cheesecake but a thin layer of plastic wrap, these pie-in-the-sky fantasies can end up setting you up for disappointment. I mean, I don't know about you, but my chances of being mistaken for any relative of Cindy Crawford are, well, slim to none. And as for being appreciated at work or having my husband grovelling at my knees or seeing my life-long nemesis,

Ms. Skinny, pack a few pounds on her washboard stomach—I don't see any of this happening any time soon!

That's why it's important to be realistic about what losing weight can—and can't—do for you. Losing can make you feel stronger, healthier, more attractive, and more in control of your eating habits. But it can't magically fix everything that's wrong with your life.

Nor will losing weight transform you into a supermodel. When you're sitting on the high side of 200 pounds, it's easy to convince yourself that every skinny person has a body that's simply to die for, but that's simply not the case. Take a look around you and you'll see what I mean: skinny people come in all shapes and sizes. They aren't all Demi Moore clones! If the truth is to be told—and frankly it's about time—there are only a handful of supermodels and Playboy bunnies among us—and a lot of them have had more than a few cosmetic surgeries to help Mother Nature along.

Bottom line? Stop dreaming in technicolour and focus instead on what losing weight can actually deliver: a slimmer (although not necessarily skinny!), healthier you.

2

The Dirt on Diets

Think dieting is a relatively recent invention — a product of the post-Twiggy, post-bikini era? Think again. Our obsession with weight loss started a good century before pencil-thin models and microscopic bathing suits led large numbers of North American women to engage in some serious navel (and thigh!) gazing.

The Not-So-Magnificent Obsession

While North Americans have been brooding about the rolls of fat around their middles for well over a hundred years, it's only been during the past few decades that dieting has tuned into a bit of an obsession.

While people flirted with the idea of losing a few extra pounds during the first few decades of the twentieth century, dieting didn't really come into vogue until the early 1950s. At that point, it began to really take off. According to Laura Fraser, author of *Losing It: False Hopes and Fat Profits in the Diet Industry*, the number of weight-loss-related articles published by women's magazines increased by 500% between 1951 and 1953 alone. (And for good reason: they were a guaranteed way of selling truckloads of magazines!) Like their modern-day counterparts, these magazine articles were typically accompanied by dramatic "before and after" photos and horrible headlines (e.g., "From forlorn fatty—to fashion model") that spelled out the dreadful fate that awaited any woman who was foolish enough to "let herself go."

As hard as these magazine articles may have been to stomach, women could still take solace in the fact that one of the hottest sex symbols of the decade—the breathless blonde starlet Marilyn Monroe—weighed in at over 150 pounds. Unfortunately, her successors in the sex symbol department weren't cut nearly the same slack. According to Nancy Etcoff, author of *Survival of the Prettiest: The Science of Beauty*, full-figured beauties like Marilyn soon found themselves on the endangered species list. Skin and bones rather than curves and padding had come into vogue:

> The Miss Americas of the 1960s were five feet six inches tall and weighed a hundred and twenty pounds. Twenty years later they had gained two inches in height but remained at the same weight. Playboy playmates also dropped several pounds and gained several inches in height during the same period, dipping from eleven percent below the national average to seventeen percent below it.

In this chapter, we're going to look at North America's obsession with weight loss. We're going to zero in on some of the worst fad diets and weight-loss products ever invented: fad diets that were so crazy, and weight-loss products that were so dangerous, that it's hard to believe anyone actually brought them to the market. Then we'll consider the reasons why so many diets—fad or not—are doomed to failure. Finally, we'll wrap up the chapter by zeroing in on proven strategies for weight-loss success—strategies that will help you to get off the dieting roller coaster once and for all.

The Fad Diet Hall of Shame

North Americans have been preoccupied with weight for well over a century. According to Laura Fraser, author of *Losing It: False Hopes and Fat Profits in the Diet Industry*, dieting first came into vogue during the 1830s, when a young Presbyterian minister named Sylvester Graham preached against the evils of overeating. He claimed that gluttony was simply the first step down the slippery slope that could lead to lust, sexual perversion, and social chaos. (The way Graham saw it, one day, you'd be sneaking into the pantry to grab a tin of biscuits; the next day, you'd be sneaking into the barn for a romp in the haystack

Food for Thought

"The worship of the willowy supermodel has become a cult, and the parent of even the scrawniest six-year-old will know that she is quite likely to come home from school announcing that she is starting a diet...."

—William Jeffcoate, M.D., of the City Hospital, in Nottingham, U.K., writing in the British medical journal *The Lancet* in 1998

Food for Thought

By 1891, public scales were being used by an increasingly weight-conscious public. A little over two decades later, the first bathroom scales hit the market. From this point forward, it would be possible to obsess about your weight in the privacy of your own home.

with whatever male happened to be handy at the time!) The solution that he served up was simple: a diet of bland food that was guaranteed to put your appetite to sleep. (Graham must have rolled over in his grave when he discovered what his descendants were up to: they were responsible for giving the world the tasty, honey-flavoured snack crackers that still bear his name today.)

The next nineteenth-century diet guru to arrive on the scene was William Banting, a British casket-maker who wrote a best-selling diet book after dropping 46 pounds from his 202-pound frame. No one seemed to think twice about buying a diet book that was put out by a casket-maker (although at least a few cynical souls must have wondered if this was his roundabout way of drumming up some additional business!): *Letter on Corpulence* managed to sell 58 000 copies before Banting's death in 1878. Unlike Graham, Banting managed to come up with a diet plan that the public was prepared to stomach: in addition to lean meat, dry toast, and soft-boiled eggs, his weight-loss plan allowed for a couple of drinks per day. (Perhaps the liquid element of the diet plan helps to explain why Banting's program was a far bigger hit in Britain than in the United States: the Americans had yet to shed their puritanical attitudes about alcohol consumption.)

The next fellow to step up to the weight-loss podium was Horace Fletcher—a turn-of-the-century weight-loss fanatic who promoted what he described as the "science" of chewing. He believed that the secret to losing weight was to chew each bite of food at least 20 times. Not only would you end up with a mouthful of food that was totally devoid of texture and taste (an effective appetite suppressant, if I've ever heard of one!), your mouth would get tired of chewing long before your stomach ever got full. The result—and Fletcher considered this to be a selling point—was that eating would become an unpleasant chore rather than something to be looked forward to and enjoyed.

Think Fletcher sounds like a bit of a flake? You haven't heard the worst yet. Apparently, Fletcher took a highly scientific approach to monitoring all aspects of his digestive functions. In addition to keeping track of the number of times he chewed his food, he made a point of weighing his feces. At one point, he went so far as to mail them to a Yale University physiologist who was studying weight reduction. (Kind of makes you wonder who was more grateful when "Fletcherism" fizzled out: the dieting public or the post office!)

Over time, the chew-your-food-to-death fad was soon replaced by another fad: not chewing anything at all. The person promoting this particular weight-loss method was none other than respected investigative journalist Upton Sinclair. He wrote an article on fasting for *Cosmopolitan* magazine in 1909, noting that not eating for days at a time left him feeling healthy and alert. (Clearly, Sinclair was the Oprah of the pre-television era: fasting clubs popped up across the U.S. shortly after the article appeared.)

Sinclair wasn't the only one with a weight-loss method to pitch at the start of the twentieth century, mind you. Around the same time, John Harvey Kellogg—future cereal magnate—took over an old nutritional sanitarium in Battle Creek, Michigan, where he offered such obesity "cures" as cold rain douches and plunge baths—proof positive, I suppose, that the cure can be worse than the disease!

Women's magazines also began to reflect this growing interest in weight-loss methods. They began carrying advertisements for a range of weight-loss products: everything from pamphlets with details about the latest wonder diet to "fat-burning" formulations of water (!) to diet pills containing thyroid. This latter product—ironically marketed under the brand name "Kellogg's Safe Fat Reducer"—caused a dieter's body to go into overdrive by speeding the thyroid up to dangerous levels. The resulting side effects included nervousness, heart palpitations, sweating, weakness, insomnia, and—in some cases—permanent damage to the nervous system.

Hard as it may be to believe, Kellogg's Safe Fat Reducer was positively healthy as compared to other diet preparations available at the time. Popular ingredients in the growing number of diet products that were available by mail order included laxatives, purgatives, washing soda, epsom salts, arsenic, dinitrophenol (a powerful insecticide and herbicide), human chorionic gonadotropin (a hormone found in the urine of pregnant women), and amphetamines. Not all weight-loss preparations were harmful, however: one highly popular product consisted of nothing other than pink lemonade!

Of course, North Americans weren't just hungry for pills to pop and diet drinks to down. Any quick fix would do! As the century marched on, they gratefully embraced all kinds of gizmos and gadgets that promised to help them lose weight. There was the Slendro Massage Table (a device that promised to jiggle off your fat), Slim-skins (inflatable rubber trousers that were attached to a vacuum cleaner), astringent body wraps and sweat-inducing rubber garments that caused dehydration, an Astro-Trimmer sauna belt that promised to take inches off your waistline, earrings that were supposed to eliminate hunger pains, and a rolling

Food for Thought

Another wacky weight-loss gadget to hit the market during the 1960s was a machine that promised to vibrate the pounds away. The theory was that the motorized canvas belt that fit around your waist would help to break up fat cells, making it easier for your body to eliminate them. All it managed to do, however, was to loosen the bills in your wallet!

pin with suction cups that was designed to help you slim down. (I haven't figured that one out yet either!)

Over time, these gadgets became increasingly high-tech. (Clearly, some of the folks working in R & D in the weight-loss industry were great fans of the gizmo-heavy children's cartoon *The Jetsons*!) No longer did you have to rely on your own sensations of hunger to decide when it was time to stop eating: the flashing green and red lights on your electric fork would do the thinking for you! And if you were tempted to grab a midnight snack before you went to bed, an electronic device on your refrigerator would tell you in no uncertain terms that you could live without the extra calories. (I kid you not. Some folks actually paid money for these contraptions.)

That Was Then, This Is Now—Right?

You'd think that by now we would have learned our lesson about fad diets and ineffective weight-loss products—that we would be far too sophisticated to fall for the same old weight-loss scams time and time again. Unfortunately, that's simply not the case. We've seen some real doozies come and go over the past thirty years:

- Liquid diets of all sorts, starting with Metrecal (the so-called "miracle diet" of the 1960s) as well as the Optifast diet that saw Oprah losing (and then regaining) 67 pounds.
- Fad diets like the Drinking Man's Diet (think martinis and steak!), as well as very low-calorie diets such as the infamous Cambridge Diet of the late 1970s, which had the less-than-desirable side effect of causing your body to feed on its own organs.
- Diets based on a single food—everything from popcorn to rice to grapefruit to cabbage soup! (The grapefruit growers were no-doubt pleased with all the talk about the so-called "fat-burning" powers of what had up until then been the Rodney Dangerfield of fruits!)

Most of us consider ourselves to be smart consumers who are capable of carefully scrutinizing the goods before we fork over our cold, hard cash, and yet it's not unusual for a North American woman to spend hundreds—even thousands—of dollars on fad diets and weight-loss-related products. (Don't think you've spent that kind of money? Grab that cheque book register and start calculating the damages for yourself. It doesn't take long for the diet books, herbal weight-loss supplements, fitness club memberships, packaged diet foods, and Weight Watchers fees to really add up.) That's why the North American weight-loss industry rings up an astounding $55 billion in sales each year!

For some reason, we seem to have a particularly big blind spot when it comes to spotting the weaknesses of the latest and greatest fad diet. We tend to forget all of the things we have ever learned about losing weight the sensible way the moment someone promises to show us a quick and painless way to make those extra pounds disappear.

We're susceptible to these types of pitches because fad diets dish up three ingredients that we find positively irresistible:

The Skinny

It's not hard to figure out why most people lose weight on single food diets—at least temporarily. After seven days of shovelling down bowl after bowl of cabbage soup or eating truckloads full of grapefruit, you're pretty much ready to gag at the sight of it.

That's not the worst news about single food diets, of course: the hardest part of all to stomach is that you tend to regain all the weight you've lost the moment you start eating normally again.

1. **Instant results (or at least the *promise* of instant results).** There's no denying it: we live in an instant society—a world in which instant everything has become the standard. (Heck, we even use instant messaging services when we're online because e-mail takes too long!) It's therefore hardly surprising at all that we want the same instant results when it comes to weight loss. Why settle for losing weight at the healthy rate of no more than one to two pounds per week when someone's offering a speedier alternative? We're always looking for a quick fix, so if a particular diet promises to help us to shed the extra pounds at lightning speed, we're ready to gamble our health and our self-esteem for a shot at rapid weight loss.

2. **An effortless method of losing weight.** If you take the sensible approach to weight loss (the approach I'm going to be spelling out at the end of this chapter), you'll have to be prepared to use your brain. You have to learn how to plan healthy meals, figure out how to squeeze trips to the gym into your insanely busy schedule, and come up with some new ways of coping with stress (as opposed to just smothering yourself with carbohydrates). All of this requires time, effort, and hard work on your part. In contrast, a fad diet can be a bit of a no-brainer. You don't have to give any thought to what you're going to pop into your mouth come dinner time (assuming, of course, that you're actually allowed to eat dinner). The diet guru du jour has already done the thinking for you. (Heck, the guru may even have done the shopping for

you, selling you a smorgasbord of diet foods that are guaranteed to help your wallet to slim down!)

3. **Hope.** The people out there flogging the latest and greatest fad diet aren't just selling you a set of menus. They're selling you hope. During those exciting first few hours when you embark on a fad diet, it's easy to convince yourself that things are going to be different this time. Forget the fact that every diet you've ever tried has failed miserably: this time you're going to end up with a fairy tale happy ending. Or at least that's what you tell yourself until the moment of truth arrives and you discover that you simply can't stomach another bowl of cabbage soup.

How to Spot a Fad Diet

Just as some women are susceptible to the wrong men, some women are susceptible to the wrong types of diets—diets that promise the earth, but don't deliver. Here are some tips on spotting fad diets before they get the chance to sweet-talk you out of your money, your health, and your self-esteem.

- Watch out for diets that make outlandish claims that seem to fly in the face of conventional nutritional wisdom. As much as you may hate to admit it to yourself, a diet that allows you to eat chocolate rather than vegetables isn't exactly based on hard scientific facts. Bottom line? Chocolate never has been and never will be a health food.
- Beware of sweet-talking diet book authors who like to wear white lab coats. It's one thing to look like a doctor: it's quite another to actually have a degree in nutrition, kinesiology, or any related discipline.
- Take all diet-related claims with a grain of salt (or an entire teaspoon, if that's what it takes!). There are no "magic" fat-burning foods, nor are there any "secrets" to lasting weight loss—other than plain, old-fashioned common sense. (Note: An eagle-eyed friend of mine,who also happens to be an eating disorders specialist, has noticed that many diet commercials contain a tiny disclaimer indicating that the results shown in the ad are not typical. So reach for your glasses the next time such an ad airs and play a quick round of "Find the Disclaimer"!)
- Be skeptical of any weight-loss program that labels certain groups of foods as "good" and certain foods as "bad." While some foods pack a bigger nutritional punch than others (a spear of broccoli wins over a pat of butter every time!), your body needs a variety of types of foods—protein, carbohydrates, and fats—in order to function properly.

- Pass on diets that promise quick and easy weight loss—more than two pounds per week. If you lose weight more rapidly than that, you end up losing a disproportionate amount of muscle—something that can cause your metabolism to nose-dive. (We'll be revisiting this issue in Chapter 4, so be sure to stay tuned!)
- Skip any program that requires you to dramatically change your eating habits in the short run, but that claims that you can go back to "eating normally" once you've lost the weight. You'll be practically dooming yourself to failure.
- Forget about any program that appears to be based on pseudoscience or quackery rather than scientific facts. There seems to be a new crop of diet quacks hitting the airwaves every week, with impressive-sounding scientific theories, but no hard evidence to substantiate their claims. More often than not, they've got products to sell, so don't be too swayed by the "free" advice that they promise to send you if you respond to their hour-long infomercials!
- Steer clear of gimmicks. The weight-loss industry is masterful at packaging the same old tired advice in sexy new ways. Don't assume that you're getting something new just because a particular program is being packaged as a diet breakthrough.
- Think twice before you decide to try a diet that's based on super-rigid menu plans or that's built around foods you would never normally eat. You could find yourself feeling frustrated because your grocery store doesn't happen to carry organically grown okra or downright horrified at the prospect of having to down a dinner of grilled tofu again! And frankly, who could blame you?
- Remind yourself that there's no such thing as a quick fix when it comes to weight loss. If a fad diet sounds too good to be true, it probably is.

The Skinny

Watch out for diet books that are high on shelf-appeal and low on substance. Celebrity diet books tend to the worst offenders, since their appeal is based more on the washboard stomach and steely thighs of the celebrity in question than any bona fide weight-loss advice that appears on the printed page.

Why Diets Don't Work

If you think there's some sort of miracle diet out there with your name on it—one that will finally take you to the promised land of slender thighs and trim hips—I've got some bad news for you, girlfriend. There's no such thing.

The sad truth is that most diets fall far short of delivering a miracle. In fact, many don't work at all. And even if a dieter does manage to beat the odds and get

Fat Chance

Think you can lose seven pounds of fat during your first week on a diet? Think again! Even if the scale drops by a full seven pounds that first week, approximately five pounds of what you've lost is water. The effect can be particularly dramatic if you go on a low-carbohydrate diet because your body is forced to draw upon its stores of carbohydrates (glycogen). Each pound of these carbohydrate stores is packed away with three to four pounds of water. Consequently, when you begin drawing upon your body's stash of glycogen, a large quantity of water is flushed from your system.

down to her ideal weight, she has—at best—a slim chance of maintaining that loss. Here's why.

The Numbers Game

The moment you go on a diet, your body switches into starvation mode. Rather than celebrating the fact that you're trying to do something about those extra pounds, it does whatever it can to hold on to them for dear life. It starts by dropping your metabolism by 15 to 30 percent within the first 24 to 48 hours of the start of your diet. (That translates into a whopping 300- to 600-calorie-per-day drop if you're used to consuming 2000 calories per day.)

If you continue to diet, but don't start exercising, your metabolism will continue to creep downward. This is because you are losing valuable muscle tissue while you're simultaneously shedding water weight and fat. Because muscle tissue burns twice as many calories as fat tissue, this drop in the amount of muscle tissue in your body can further decrease the number of calories that you need in a day in order to maintain your weight—something that can slow your weight loss or, even worse, make it easy for you to regain the weight that you've lost. The only way around this metabolic tug of war is to exercise while you're losing weight (to offset as much of the loss of muscle tissue as possible) and to lose weight slowly (to avoid throwing your body into starvation mode).

Food Cravings: Friend or Foe?

Just in case your body can't maintain your weight by fiddling with your metabolism, it has another weapon in its anti-starvation arsenal: food cravings!

Think you're the only one struggling with food cravings? You're actually in very good company. A recent study showed that 97

The Skinny

There are few issues as hotly debated in the weight-loss community as what constitutes a "safe" rate of weight loss. Some experts argue that you should aim for a rate of no more than half a pound a week. Others, however, feel that this rate of weight loss is too discouraging for anyone other than that rare dieter who is genetically programmed to have the patience of a saint! The standard party line these days seems to be that a weight loss of one to two pounds a week is ideal: it's speedy enough to give you impressive results, but not so sudden that your metabolism hits the panic button.

percent of women and 69 percent of men experience food cravings on a regular basis. (Chocolate is the most craved food for about 50 percent of women and 15 percent of men.)

As hard as they can be to contend with, cravings are actually a sensible reaction to dieting. Consider what registered dietitian Debra Waterhouse had to say about them in a recent issue of *PMS Access*—a U.S. health newsletter:

> In the past, food cravings were viewed as a sign of weakness, something we had to find the willpower deep in the soul to overcome. In fact, it's to our benefit to trust our bodies and appreciate the food messages they're giving us.

The message that these cravings are trying to give you, of course, is that you've cut back your food intake too drastically. Cravings are your body's way of sending an SOS to your brain—an SOS that says, "Feed me now!"

The Psychological Fallout of Dieting

As if metabolic shifts, food cravings, and the other physical effects of dieting weren't enough for a dieter to contend with, there is also the psychological fall-out to be considered. Dieting can be stressful—so stressful, indeed, that at least one study blames it for damaging the body's immune system!

Immune system consequences aside, most experts agree that dieting fosters an unhealthy relationship with food. It teaches you to treat some foods as "good" and some foods as "bad"—something that can set you up for a major M & Ms binge when you get sick of indulging in "good" foods like cottage cheese and melba toast. (As Geneen Roth notes in her book *When You Eat at the Refrigerator, Pull Up a Chair*, "For every diet, there is an equal and opposite binge.")

Dieting also teaches you to feel bad about yourself if you happen to fall off the wagon—and chances are you ultimately will. Unfortunately, some dieters feel so bad about themselves when this happens that they never manage to get back on the wagon again.

The Skinny

Wondering how to cope with food cravings? According to Janis Jibrin, author of *The Unofficial Guide to Dieting Safely*, behaviour modification is the key. She suggests that you start trying to cut back on the number of times you give in to your cravings and the amount you consume each time you succumb. Try having one scoop of ice cream rather than two, and make an effort to have the odd treat-free day, too. Don't try to make too many changes too quickly, however; she cautions: "A carrot stick isn't going to cut it when you feel like Godiva, so have a little piece of chocolate."

The Skinny

Some experts believe that the physical and emotional stress of dieting can damage your immune system, leaving you more susceptible to disease.

That's certainly been my pattern over the years, I must confess. Like any Type A++ personality, I like to achieve and I hate to fail. When I'm "on a diet," I tend to follow the program to the tee—weighing my tuna, carefully measuring my low-fat mayo, and eating two-thirds of a slice of bread rather than the whole slice if that's all my one ounce serving from the bread group will "buy" me.

Unfortunately, you can't live like that forever. At some point, you're going to have to allow yourself to live a little—and that's where I've traditionally run into trouble. I have vivid memories, for example, of how I lost control on Christmas Day of 1978. After months of going to Weight Watchers and getting down to a svelte-for-me 135 pounds, I found myself alone in the kitchen with platter after platter of mouth-watering food. At first I was seduced by a bran muffin—a warm, butter-glistened homemade type that was full of plump, juicy raisins. Then it was a couple of Nanaimo bars: after all, if I'd blown the diet by having that bran muffin, there didn't seem to be much point in holding back now. Soon I was inhaling every forbidden food in sight: gingerbread cookies, shortbreads, candy canes, and chocolate Santas. The diet was officially over.

The Solution

It's obvious that dieting isn't the answer if you're serious about losing weight and keeping it off. So what is the solution?

Most experts agree that there is only one way to shed the pounds and banish them for good—and it's a two-for-one deal. Not only do you have to make some permanent changes to your eating habits: you also have to commit to exercising on a regular basis.

I admit it: it isn't the sexiest solution. You were probably hoping that I'd uncovered some new study about the metabolism-boosting powers of chocolate! All kidding aside, however, this particular double whammy gives you the greatest odds of losing the extra weight once and for all. Exercise is the "secret ingredient" that so many weight-loss programs have been missing over the years.

It isn't difficult to figure out why exercise can help you to lose weight. For one thing, it helps you to burn off fat—and, as you've no doubt discovered by now, it's pretty hard to lose weight just by cutting back on the amount of food you eat.

(You have to burn off an extra 3500 calories in order to lose a single pound. That works out to an entire week of burning off 500 more calories less each day than what you take in.) Bottom line? Unless you have the willpower of a saint and/or an appetite that can be turned on and off at will, you'll probably find that it's a whole lot easier to burn off at least some of the fat through exercise than to rely on calorie-cutting alone.

There are, of course, a couple of added bonuses to exercising while you lose weight: exercise can play a powerful role in jump-starting even the most sluggish metabolism and it can help your body to build muscle tissue—something that can help to make up for any muscle tissue that's being lost as the pounds start coming off. We'll be returning to this issue again in Chapter 4, "Gym Class Revisited." But first, let's hit the kitchen for a crash course in nutrition.

The Skinny

Your body needs about 10 calories per day for each pound of body weight in order to keep you alive. (Hey, it takes energy to keep the blood circulating and the air pumping through your lungs!) That means that a 200-pound woman has a basal metabolic rate of approximately 2000 calories. Since your body requires an extra 10 percent of calories just to digest your food and an extra 30 percent to fuel physical activity (assuming that you're at least moderately active), a 200-pound woman needs about 2800 calories per day in order to maintain her weight. If she drops that calorie intake to 2300 calories, she can expect to lose about a pound a week. If she drops it to 1800 calories, she can expect to lose about two pounds per week.

3

A Recipe for Success

Trying to stick to an "off-the-shelf" diet plan is like trying to squeeze into a pair of one-size-fits-all pantyhose: the odds of ending up with a comfortable fit are pretty much slim to none!

If you've had less-than-stellar results from diets that appear to have been designed for high-flying Hollywood celebrities who can afford such frills as personal chefs and live-in fitness trainers rather than for average folks like you and me, you may be ready to try something different.

That's exactly what I'm proposing. Rather than trying your luck at another round of diet roulette—gambling that you'll end up with an off-the-shelf diet plan that you can actually stick with for more than a week!—why not try designing your own weight-loss program this time around?

As crazy as this idea may sound (and it may sound downright insane to you if you're someone who is used putting your fate in the hands of the latest—but not necessarily greatest—weight-loss gurus), a do-it-yourself weight-loss program actually makes a lot of sense. After all, who other than you is better equipped to design a weight-loss program that will take into account your overbooked schedule, your one-of-a-kind food preferences, and the thousand-and-one other things that have short-circuited your past attempts at losing weight?

I'm not the only one who's convinced of the merits of do-it-yourself weight-loss programs, by the way. A lot of the big-name obesity researchers are also singing the praises of these types of programs—and for good reason: there's a growing body of evidence to show that do-it-yourself weight-loss programs tend to be a lot more successful than their off-the-shelf counterparts.

It's not that difficult to figure out why. You learn a lot more when you accept responsibility for designing your own weight-loss program than if you go into lemming mode and follow someone else's. (Didn't lose any weight the first week on Dr. Slim's Amazing Cheesecake Diet? No problem! You can always blame it on Dr. Slim. Didn't lose any weight on your do-it-yourself program? The buck stops with you, honey. It's back to the drawing board!)

Food for Thought

Ignorance isn't necessarily bliss when it comes to weight loss. A recent study at New York-based Niagara University revealed that people who hold irrational beliefs about food (e.g., "calories don't count if food is eaten while standing") were more likely to have weight problems than their more food-savvy (and smarter!) peers.

Designing a Program That Will Work for You

Not sure how to go about designing a weight-loss program? There's no need to hit the panic button yet. Contrary to what you might think, you don't have to reinvent the wheel: you can cheat by begging, borrowing, and stealing bits and pieces from weight-loss programs that have worked well for you in the past.

Here are some points to consider when you're evaluating past weight-loss efforts and trying to map out a strategy that will ensure your future success:

- What types of weight-loss programs have worked well for you in the past? What was it about these programs that seemed to work well? Would they still work for you at this point in your life? Why or why not?
- What types of weight-loss programs haven't worked well for you in the past? What was it about these programs that didn't work well for you? What would have made the plan work better for you?
- Do you tend to be more successful when you're following a very rigid eating program or one that's a bit more flexible?
- Are you someone who needs group or one-on-one support? If so, how will you factor this into your weight-loss program? (Note: You'll find plenty of tips on getting the support you need in Chapter 6, "Sister Act.")
- Do you have a lot of time to devote to shopping and food preparation? If not, how will you work around this limitation when you're designing your own weight-loss program?
- Have you had difficulty maintaining previous weight losses? What went wrong? How will you avoid this problem this time around?
- How will you fit exercise into your program? (Note: You'll find plenty of information on getting active in Chapter 4, "Gym Class Revisited.")

Food for Thought

Here's something to chew on the next time you hit the all-you-can-eat buffet: researchers believe that one of the keys to living a longer life is eating less. Rats who were fed 40% fewer calories than other rats lived one-third longer than rats who were allowed to eat as much as they wanted.

- What recommendations (if any) has your doctor made concerning your exercise and weight-loss plans?

If you haven't had a lot of success with previous efforts to lose weight, you might want to consider using *Canada's Food Guide to Healthy Eating* (see Table 3.1) as the basic blueprint for your do-it-yourself weight-loss program. Frankly, it's as good a starting point as any because it's based on sound nutritional principles. What's more, since it's such a flexible eating plan—it's designed to meet the needs of everyone from a 50-pound preschooler to a 300-pound football player!—you won't have much difficulty customizing this eating program to meet your own nutritional needs and lifestyle. (Note: The U.S. *Food Pyramid* is very similar to Canada's *Food Guide to Healthy Eating*. It's also based on sound nutritional principles. If you're more familiar with the *Food Pyramid* than our own home-grown *Food Guide*, you might want to design your weight-loss program around it instead.)

Of course, if you decide to eat the maximum number of servings that the *Food Guide* allows, you could find yourself in weight-gain rather than weight-loss mode! (Don't forget: this plan is designed to meet the nutritional needs of Canadians of all shapes and sizes, not just people who are hoping to lose weight.) You can, however, easily turn the *Food Guide* into a blueprint for weight-loss success. Here's how:

- Limit the number of servings that you consume each day from each of the four major food groups. Rather than wolfing down a dozen slices of bread each day just because the *Food Guide* says you're "allowed" twelve servings, cut your consumption to five servings instead. (If you're still hungry, try adding servings from the vegetables, fruit and grain products groups before adding back servings from the remaining food groups. You may have to fiddle with the number of servings until you stumble upon the quantity that's just right for you—enough to ensure that you feel satisfied, but not so much that your weight-loss grinds to a halt. If you go with the minimum number of servings for each food group, you'll be consuming about 1800 calories per day, depending on the types of food choices you make within each food group.)
- Emphasize cereals, breads, other grain products, vegetables, and fruit when you're planning your menus. They tend to be lower in fat—and therefore

TABLE 3.1

CANADA'S FOOD GUIDE TO HEALTHY EATING

Canada's Food Guide to Healthy Eating is designed to provide you with an adequate number of servings from each of the four basic food groups: grain products, vegetables and fruit, milk products, and meat and alternatives.

FOOD GROUP	WHY YOU NEED THIS TYPE OF FOOD	NUMBER OF SERVINGS YOU NEED IN A DAY	WHAT CONSTITUTES A SERVING
Grain products	Grain products are critical for converting food to energy and for maintaining a healthy nervous system. They are also an excellent source of B vitamins.	5 to 12 servings	• 1 slice of bread • 30 grams (one ounce) of cold cereal • 175 ml (3/4 cup) of hot cereal • 1/2 a bagel, pita, or bun • 125 ml (1/2 cup) of pasta or rice
Vegetables and fruit	Vegetables and fruits are a good source of fibre and an excellent source of vitamins A and C, as well as hundreds of disease-fighting compounds called phyto-chemicals.	5 to 10 servings	• 1 medium-sized vegetable or fruit • 125 ml (1/2 cup) fresh, frozen, or canned vegetables or fruit • 250 ml (1 cup) of tossed salad • 125 ml (1/2 cup) of fruit juice
Milk products	Milk products are an excellent source of calcium, the mineral that is responsible for keeping our bones healthy and strong and staving off osteoporosis, a debilitating bone-thinning disease.	2 to 4 servings	• 250 ml (one cup) milk • 50 grams (approximately 1-1/2 ounces) of hard cheese • 175 ml (3/4 cup) of yogurt
Meat and alternatives	Meat and alternatives provide excellent sources of protein, iron, and zinc.	2 to 3 servings	• 50 grams to 100 grams (1-1/2 ounces to 3 ounces) of meat, poultry, or fish • one to two eggs • 125 ml to 250 ml (1/2 cup to one cup) of beans • 100 grams (3 ounces) of tofu • 30 ml (2 tbsp.) of peanut butter

Note: *Canada's Food Guide to Healthy Eating* also makes mention of "other foods"—foods and beverages that aren't part of any other food group. They include foods that are mostly fats and oils, such as butter, margarine, cooking oil, and lard; foods that are mostly sugar, such as jam, honey, syrup, and candies; high-fat and/or high-salt snack foods such as chips (potato, corn, etc.) or pretzels; beverages such as water, tea, coffee, alcohol, and soft drinks; and herbs, spices, and condiments such as pickles, mustard, and ketchup. Some of these foods, like water, should be enjoyed often; others, like snack foods and alcohol, should be used in moderation.

Sources: *Canada's Food Guide to Healthy Eating*. Ottawa: Health and Welfare Canada, 1992. *The Unofficial Guide to Dieting Safely* by Janis Jibrin. New York: IDG Books, 1998.

The Skinny

Want to kiss those extra pounds goodbye for good? A low-fat, low-calorie diet appears to be your best option. Researchers at the National Weight Control Registry have discovered that the weight-loss program of choice for individuals who have maintained weight losses of at least 30 pounds for five years or longer is a low-fat, low-calorie diet.

lower in calories—than foods in the milk products and meat and alternatives groups. (While protein and carbohydrates contain just four calories per gram, a gram of fat carries a button-popping nine calories per gram. Hey, it's no wonder they call it fat!)

• Try to make the healthiest possible choices when you're selecting foods from of the four major food groups. Choose foods that pack as much of a nutritional punch as possible so that you can ensure that your body gets the best "buy" for its caloric "dollar." (Just in case you dozed off in Grade 8 home economics class, I've summarized the most important facts about vitamins and minerals in Table 3.2.)

TABLE 3.2

FROM A TO ZINC: THE NUTRIENTS YOUR BODY NEEDS

WHAT IT IS	WHAT IT DOES	WHERE TO FIND IT
Vitamin A (retinol and carotene)	Maintains skin and body tissues and plays a role in vision. Helps your body to respond to infection. May help to reduce the risk of lung cancer.	Liver, fortified milk, carrots, tomatoes, cantaloupe, whole milk, butter, cheese, egg yolk, cod, and other fatty fish
Beta-carotene (a plant pigment that our bodies convert to vitamin A as needed)	Believed to help to reduce the risk of cancer and heart disease in non-smokers.	Orange-fleshed vegetables such as carrots, yams, and butternut squash; dark leafy greens such as kale and broccoli; cantaloupe and papaya
Vitamin B1 (thiamine)	Helps your body to convert carbo-hydrates into energy. Necessary for the proper functioning of the nervous system.	Whole grains, enriched grains, legumes, nuts, beans, organ meats, pork, brewer's yeast, wheat germ
Vitamin B2 (riboflavin)	Promotes tissue growth and regen-eration and enables your body to use carbohydrates, fat, and protein. Aids in adrenal function	Brewer's yeast, wheat germ, whole grains, green leafy vegetables, milk, cheese, other milk products, eggs
Vitamin B3 (niacin)	Helps to release energy from food and plays a role in both DNA synthesis and the maintenance of healthy skin, nerves, and digestive processes.	Whole grains, wheat germ, organ meats, green vegetables, oily fish, eggs, milk, poultry, cereal, legumes
Vitamin B5 (pantothenic acid)	Aids in the metabolism of food, especially protein. Helps to stabilize blood sugar levels and to synthesize antibodies, cholesterol, hemoglobin, and some hormones.	Organ meats, eggs, peanuts, cheese, cereals, milk, vegetables

Vitamin B6 (pyridoxine)	Enables your body to make use of protein. Also asists in metabolism of carbohydrates. Plays a role in proper nerve function and synthesis of red blood cells.	Brewer's yeast, whole grains, soy flour, organ meats, wheat germ, mushrooms, potatoes
Vitamin B12 (cyanocobalamin)	Used to form hemoglobin. Helps your body to make use of protein, folic acid, and fatty acids.	Kidney, fish, milk, eggs, meat
Vitamin C (ascorbic acid)	Helps with the formation of connective tissue and the absorption of iron. Assists with both healing and the formation of healthy bones. Helps control blood cholesterol.	Citrus fruits, strawberries, dark-green leafy vegetables, and tomatoes
Vitamin D (calciferol)	Helps to keep your bones healthy. Necessary for calcium absorption.	Fortified milk, oily fish, eggs, butter, liver
Vitamin E	A potent antioxidant. Helps to protect cells from damage and degeneration. Maintains muscles and red blood cells.	Wheat germ, egg yolks, peanuts, seeds, vegetable oils
Vitamin K	Aids in blood coagulation.	Leafy green vegetables
Boron	Helps your body to retain calcium and magnesium and may play a role in preserving bone.	Fruits and vegetables
Calcium	Strengthens bones and teeth, promotes blood clotting, and regulates nerve and muscle function and metabolism.	Milk, cheese, sardines, salmon, oysters, shrimp, tofu, kale, and broccoli
Choline	Plays an important role in the maintenance of cells and in transporting fats throughout the body.	Milk, eggs, peanuts
Chromium	Critical to the proper functioning of insulin—the hormone that helps to regulate blood sugar. Works with insulin to metabolize glucose.	Meat, whole-grain breads and cereals, wheat germ, and orange juice
Copper	Helps your body to use iron and aids in energy metabolism.	Chicken, fish, meat avocados, potatoes, soybeans, nuts, seeds
Folic acid	Assists with cell division. A critical nutrient prior to and during pregnancy. Helps to synthesize amino acids.	Raw leafy vegetables, soy flour, oranges, bananas, walnuts, brewer's yeast, legumes
Iodine	Necessary to make thyroid hormones.	Iodized table salt, shellfish, seaweed
Iron	Necessary for the formation of red blood cells, which carry oxygen to your tissues. Helps to prevent iron-deficiency anemia.	Kidneys, fish, egg yolks, red meat, cereals, molasses, apricot, shellfish, dried fruits

Magnesium	Teams up with calcium to help build bone. Aids in muscle contraction and relaxation and plays a role in energy metabolism, blood sugar regulation, nerve transmission, and in eliminating waste products from the body.	Low-fat milk, peanuts, bananas, wheat germ, dark-green leafy vegetables, oysters, tofu, and some fish
Manganese	Part of many enzyme systems. Essential for normal growth and bone formation.	Whole grains and fruits and vegetables
Molybdenum	Component of enzymes required for metabolism. Aids in iron storage.	Milk, beans, whole grains
Phosphorus	Helps to generate energy in cells. Plays a major role in bone and teeth health and DNA. Essential for proper metabolism.	Milk and milk products, meat, poultry, fish, whole-grain cereals, legumes
Potassium	Helps to maintain proper muscle tone and fluid balance.	Fruits, vegetables, fish, peanuts, potatoes
Selenium	Strengthens the immune system. Works with vitamin E to protect cell membranes from oxidative damage.	Whole grains, seafood, lean meat
Zinc	Strengthens the enzymes that drive the metabolic system. Necessary for the production of insulin.	Wheat bran, eggs, nuts, onions, shellfish, sunflower seeds, wheat germ, whole wheat, lean meat, turkey, dried beans and peas

Sources: *Canada's Food Guide to Healthy Eating.* Ottawa: Health and Welfare Canada, 1992. *The Unofficial Guide to Dieting Safely* by Janis Jibrin. New York: IDG Books, 1998. *Foods That Harm, Foods That Heal: An A to Z Guide to Safe and Healthy Eating.* Montreal: Reader's Digest, 1996. *The Unofficial Guide to Having a Baby* by Ann Douglas and John R. Sussman, M.D. IDG Books, 1999.

Food for Thought

A recent study conducted at Purdue University in Indiana revealed that calcium may act as a roadblock in the fat storage process, preventing excess calories from migrating to your thighs. According to researcher Dorothy Teegarden, who shared her tips with *Runner's World*, women who boost their calcium intake to 1000 mg per day could find themselves dropping an extra seven pounds over the next two years. Of course, this is just one study, so stay tuned for further research on this front.

Using an Off-the-Shelf Weight-Loss Program

Of course, there's nothing wrong with using an off-the-shelf weight-loss program, provided that it's nutritionally sound and it seems to be a good fit for you.

Here are some questions that you'll want to ask when you're evaluating the merits of a particular diet plan or commercial weight-loss program:

- **Is it healthy?** If it bears only a passing resemblance to *Canada's Food Guide to Healthy Eating*, it's probably not your best bet.

- **Does it provide at least 1200 calories per day?** If your calorie level drops much below this, your body will go into starvation mode and put the brakes on your metabolism.

- **Does it advocate a healthy rate of weight loss?** If the plan promises to deliver a weight loss of more than two pounds per week, it's probably too low in calories.
- **Does it place certain foods off limits?** Diets based on single foods or that suggest that you lay off entire categories of foods (e.g., dairy products or wheat) are not only hard to stick with, they're also downright unhealthy.
- **Does it include an exercise plan?** It should. A growing body of evidence is proving that dieting and exercise have to go hand in hand.
- **Does it require that you purchase special supplements such as herbs, amino acids, or vitamins and minerals or specially packaged diet foods?** You could end up getting little, if any, value for your money, so go in with your eyes wide open.
- **Does it make outlandish claims that don't stand up to scrutiny?** Remember, there's no quick fix for obesity.
- **Was the program designed by qualified people with an appropriate nutritional background?** The last thing you need is a program designed by some quack!
- **Is it suitable for everyone, regardless of their health and their weight?** As we noted earlier, there's no such thing as a one-size-fits-all weight-loss program.
- **Is it designed to help modify your eating habits, exercise patterns, and/or ways of coping with stress?** These are skills you will need to develop if you're going to maintain your weight loss successfully.
- **Is there a maintenance phase built into the program?** It's one thing to lose the weight; it's quite another to keep it off.
- **Does it sound like the right program for you?** There's no point signing up if you can't make the weekly meetings or you can't afford the specialty foods that are required as part of the food plan.

The Skinny

The top six weight-loss program red flags, according to Janis Jibrin, R.D., author of *The Unofficial Guide to Dieting Safely*:

1. You are required to purchase herbal and/or or vitamin/mineral supplements.
2. Hair and blood tests are used to measure nutritional deficiencies—one of the hottest scams in the weight-loss industry these days.
3. Certain categories of food are forbidden entirely or the program is based on a nutritionally unsound fad diet.
4. The program is less-than-upfront when it comes to hidden costs and program fees.
5. No health care professionals have been involved in designing the program.
6. The program promotes rapid weight loss (e.g., more than two pounds per week, unless it's a medically supervised diet).

The Skinny

It's pretty tedious to have to place every morsel of food on to a food scale or into a measuring cup before it touches your lips. You can eliminate the need to measure the same foods over and over again by figuring out how much food your favourite cups and dishes hold. Once you figure out that the bowls that came with your set of dishes are capable of holding a cup-and-a-half of food, you'll never have to reach for the dreaded measuring cup again!

Winning Ways

Determined to win the Battle of the Bulge once and for all? Here are some sure-fire tips for designing a bullet-proof weight-loss program:

- Don't fall prey to Mother Hubbard syndrome. Go shopping before your cupboards get too bare. If you get in the habit of keeping a variety of healthy foods on hand, you'll always have the makings of a meal. That could save you an emergency phone call to the local pizza joint—and consequently a lot of cash and calories!
- Learn how to size up the enemy. Portion control can play a huge role in making or breaking a weight-loss program. In fact, one study reported in the *New England Journal of Medicine* revealed that many overweight people underestimate portion sizes by as much as 50 percent! Bottom line? If you're not sure whether the serving of yogurt you're about to eat is a half cup or a whole cup, stop and measure. Your thighs will thank you for it!
- Eat slowly. Studies have shown that it takes about 20 minutes for your body to realize that it's full (something that goes a long way to explaining why your appetizer can leave you feeling full by the time your entrée arrives). If you hoover your dinner at record-breaking speeds, you will end up consuming far more calories than your body needs by the time the "full" sign starts flashing in your brain. A better alternative is to eat slowly so that your brain will have the chance to tell your stomach when it's time to put on the brakes.
- Bulk up. I'm not talking about bulking up your muscles à la Arnold Schwarzenegger, but rather adding more bulk to your diet. Choosing bulky, low-fat foods like fruits, vegetables, and whole-grain breads will allow you to feel full or satisfied more of the time—something that will make it easier for you to stick with your weight-loss program.
- Treat your dinner plate like an artist's canvas. Design your meals for maximum impact. Be sure to consider both eye appeal and tongue appeal when you're planning your menu. Learn how to incorporate foods of a variety of colours, shapes, textures, temperatures, and flavours into each and every meal. Who says you have to suffer because you're trying to lose weight? Indulge, indulge, indulge!

- Don't allow yourself to get caught in a rut. Rather than eating the same tired old foods for breakfast, lunch, and dinner—a trap that all too many dieters fall into—allow yourself to live a little. Experiment with foods and cooking methods that you've never tried before. Pick up some spices you've never even heard of and see what they taste like on a plate of grilled veggies. Do whatever it takes to add variety to your food choices. After all, the more fun you have with your food plan, the more likely you will be to stick with it.

- Develop a fear of frying. Choose baked and broiled foods over their fried counterparts and you'll save yourself plenty of unnecessary calories. (If you can't bear to part ways with your frying pan, you can whip yourself up a meal with the same great taste by cooking with non-fat cooking spray and ample doses of spices.)

- Tame the fat monster. Look for painless ways to trim your fat intake. Buy low-fat or no-fat salad dressing, sour cream, and dairy products. The results can be quite dramatic: If you get in the habit of using fat-free evaporated milk rather than cream in your coffee, you'll save yourself half the calories—something that could add up to a hundred calories per day or a mind-boggling 36 500 calories per year if you're someone who likes her java!

- Convince yourself to pass on those oh-so-tempting extras like butter, margarine, and regular salad dressing by considering what other types of foods those high-fat calories could buy you instead. If you leave that pat of butter on the serving plate, you could save yourself enough calories to indulge in a whole-grain roll or a small piece of fruit instead. There's just one small caveat that I need to add here: don't cut out butter completely if you'll feel deprived without it or if you'll be tempted to binge on it later on. (This is definitely one of those situations in which an ounce of prevention is worth a pound of cure!)

Fat Chance

Think that skipping breakfast will help you to lose weight? Think again. Not only are you more likely to make up for those lost calories later in the day — studies have shown that breakfast skippers have metabolic rates that are 4% to 5% lower than normal.

If you've been skipping breakfast because you don't feel hungry in the morning, here's some good news: you can train your body to feel hungry at the appropriate time by going light on your evening meal and skipping the midnight snack. Then, by the time morning rolls around, you'll be ready to hit the refrigerator.

The Skinny

Looking for a low-fat alternative to sour cream on your baked potato? Try topping it with salsa instead. (If you can't live without the creamy texture of sour cream, throw in a couple of tablespoons of yogurt, too.)

Food for Thought

Foods that are high in fat cause your circulation to slow down, reducing the oxygen-carrying capacity of the red blood cells. That's why you feel downright sluggish after eating a meal that's high in fat.

- Don't go cold turkey when it comes to cutting out high-fat foods. Change your eating habits gradually. If you move too quickly, your taste buds will orchestrate a mutiny!
- Experiment with lower-fat ways of cooking and baking. Sauté vegetables in a small amount of white wine rather than cooking them in vegetable oil. Use puréed cottage cheese instead of sour cream when you're cooking or baking. And replace some of the oil in muffins and other baked goods with unsweetened applesauce. Fortunately, there are a number of excellent cookbooks that can help you to make the transition to low-fat cooking. (You'll find my favourites listed in Appendix E.)
- Start seeing other vegetables. Rather than hanging out with the same old dinner companions, invite a new vegetable over for a change. Better yet, join the "Veggie of the Month Club": promise yourself that you'll try at least one new vegetable each month.
- Find creative ways to sneak veggies into your diet. Add cooked carrots to a bowl of low-fat chicken noodle soup or purée them and use them as a thickener in your homemade spaghetti sauce. (This is a great way to up your veggie intake if you're not exactly a card-carrying member of the Vegetable Appreciation Society.)

Fat Chance

Think all calories are created equal? Think again! According to obesity researcher James O. Hill of the University of Colorado Health Sciences Center, 90% of excess calories from fat but just 70% of excess calories from carbohydrates are converted into body fat. The reason is simple: it takes less effort for your body to convert fat to body fat than to turn carbohydrates into body fat. This means that you'll lose weight more quickly by following a low-fat, low-calorie diet than by following a high-fat, low-calorie diet.

- Give your salad a promotion. Instead of treating it as an understudy to the main dish, give it star billing. Top a leafy green salad with chicken, low-fat cheese, and some vegetable sticks and you'll end up with a healthy and delicious meal in less time that it would take for a bag of grease-drenched Chinese food to show up at your door.
- Don't be afraid to buy pre-made salads, peeled baby carrots, and pre-chopped stir-fry veggies. They may cost a little more than other produce, but they're generally worth every penny. (How often have you thrown an entire grocery bag full of salad ingredients into the compost because you were too busy to peel and chop them? Face it: those vegetables weren't any bargain!)

- Get in the habit of having a piece of fruit with each meal. It's an excellent way to fill yourself up and ensure that you're getting a variety of important nutrients. Try adding fresh or canned fruit (juice packed, of course!) to your cereal in the morning and having a serving of fruit for dessert at both lunch and dinner.
- Bring a piece of fruit and a serving of vegetables with you to work. They make a much healthier alternative to the chocolate bar vending machine! (Hint: You can make it easier for yourself to enjoy messy fruits like oranges and pears on the job if you keep a box of baby wipes in your desk.)
- Keep a container full of chopped veggies in your refrigerator and a fruit bowl on your kitchen counter. That way, you'll always have a healthy alternative to junk food. (Hint: You can dress up your veggies with a dip made of puréed black beans and spices and you can create your own fruit dipping sauce by grating some orange peel into a couple of tablespoons of low-fat yogurt.)
- Learn the "grain" truth. Find creative ways to increase your intake of whole-grain foods. They're not just healthier. They leave you feeling full longer because they take longer to digest and they keep your blood sugar on an even kilter, something that can help to prevent the post-mealtime energy dip that many people experience. Switch from white bread to whole wheat bread. Try grains you've never had before, like barley, bulgur, and oat bran. Use a mix of whole-wheat flour and white flour when you're baking. And ditch the white rice and plain pasta in favour of brown rice and whole wheat pasta.
- If you find that eating carbohydrates on their own leaves you feeling hungry afterward, try teaming your carbs up with a course of protein. Eating protein and carbohydrates at the same time allows the carbohydrates to break down into sugar at a slower rate, giving you more sustained energy and preventing those dreadful blood sugar swings that can have you sprinting toward the closest vending

The Skinny

If cooked vegetables leave you cold, perhaps it's time to rethink your cooking method. Try roasting or grilling your veggies instead of steaming or boiling them. Just marinate them in low-fat dressing or sprinkle them with spices and then bake them in the oven at 400°F for 15 minutes. Voila! You'll never look at cooked vegetables the same way again.

Food for Thought

Is it possible to be addicted to chocolate? According to a recent study in the *International Journal of Eating Disorders*, yes! Researchers in Finland found that "chocolate addicts" exhibit the same types of addictive behaviours as other types of addicts—powerful cravings and out-of-control behaviour.

machine. Carbohydrates and protein make an almost unbeatable team—the ultimate in appetite suppressants!

- When you're shopping around for a worthy carbohydrate to devour, think high fibre. New research shows that low-fibre diets may actually promote weight gain by increasing your appetite and making it easier for your body to store rather than burn fat.
- Put meat in its place. Rather than giving meat the star treatment at the dinner table, treat it as a side dish or a condiment. (As a rule of thumb, a typical serving of meat, chicken, or fish shouldn't be any larger than a deck of cards.)
- Choose the leanest possible sources of protein: poultry, fish, peas, beans, lentils, lean cuts of meat, and low-fat dairy products. There's no reason to cut beef out of your diet entirely, by the way: today's beef is 35% leaner than it was just 15 years ago.

There you have it: the ingredients for a healthy eating plan! Now let's move on and consider the flip side of the coin—your exercise program.

4

Gym Class Revisited

Looking for the secret to permanent weight loss? Forget about forking over your hard-earned cash for some high-priced "miracle cure" that comes in a jar. The answer to your weight-loss prayers is something a heck of a lot cheaper and a whole lot less gimmicky. What I'm talking about, of course, is nothing other than the dreaded e-word itself: exercise!

I know, I know. Exercise isn't exactly your favourite thing in the world. It's not mine either. I mean, given the choice between spending an afternoon at the gym or lounging on the couch reading novels, I'd definitely succumb to the magnetic pull of the couch. (Of course, this is all pie-in-the-sky stuff: the chances of me getting an afternoon to do anything other than chase after my four kids is slim to zero!) Anyway, what I'm trying to tell you is that you might want to force yourself to read this chapter, even if you're convinced that the word "exercise" is merely a euphemism for "torture."

As you've probably gathered by now, this chapter approaches the topic of exercise in a rather unconventional way. You see, rather than pretending that I go into fits of rapture each time I step on the treadmill at the gym or trying to convince you that I live for those rare stolen moments on the Stairmaster, I'm going to tell it like it is.

Exercise, to me, is a necessary evil: something I do because it's good for me, not because it's my idea of a fun way to spend an hour or two. Yes, I feel a whole lot better when I exercise—just as my mouth feels a whole lot better when I floss my teeth. That doesn't mean that I hop out of bed and eagerly dash over to my

Food for Thought

dental floss dispenser each morning, however—nor does it mean that I can't wait to hop on my exercise bike each night.

Even though exercising might not be my absolute favourite thing to do, I know that I feel better when I'm active. I feel more energetic and more alive. I also know that I don't ever want to go back to the way I was a year-and-a-half ago, when I was still a card-carrying member of the International Order of Couch Potatoes: someone who got winded carrying a basket of laundry up a flight of stairs and who had yet to recognize the joy that can come from being physically active.

Yes, I admit it: there is joy to be had from moving your body. Most of the time, you experience it when your workout is finished—when you stop and reflect upon what you've just managed to accomplish. But sometimes you experience it in the middle of a workout—when it suddenly dawns on you that you've just set a new record for yourself on the treadmill or the exercise bike. (Whenever that happens, I swear I can hear the theme from *Rocky* playing in my head!)

In this chapter, we're going to talk about the joys of being physically active: what you stand to gain health-wise by getting your body in motion and what you need to know to design the ultimate workout for yourself. But first, we're going to start out by talking about a subject that most fitness books choose to ignore: why so many women hate exercise.

Why So Many Women Hate to Exercise

Like many women who grew up in the sixties and seventies, I spent my formative years trying to avoid gym class. Hanging out in the nurse's room and pretending to be ill seemed a small price to pay for getting to sit out the sport du jour, be it volleyball, track and field, or (groan!) gymnastics. Almost 30 years after the fact, I can still remember the joy of finding out that I had to miss my public school's annual track and field day because my eye was on the mend following surgery. (Yes, the surgery was unpleasant, but anything that spared me the humiliation of being the last kid picked for track and field teams for the umpteenth year in a row couldn't be all bad!)

Yes, I still have flashbacks about gym class from time to time—and for good reason, too, I might add! I mean, we're talking cruel and usual punishment here. One of the most humiliating moments in my entire childhood happened in gym class. I can still remember what I was wearing at the time—a bright red body suit. (Just in case you've managed to repress your own gym class memories, allow me remind you what body suits were all about. They were basically one-piece bathing suits, but they suffered from a fatal design flaw: they snapped at the crotch.) Now I suppose if you purchased a high-end body suit—the kind that gymnasts wear, for example—a body suit would be a sensible enough thing to wear to gym class. Unfortunately, the one that my mother ordered for me from the Eaton's catalogue was a substandard model. As if it weren't bad enough that the body suit in question made my chunky little body look like a giant M & M: those blasted crotch snaps popped open during a particularly robust game of volleyball—the first and only time I ever put heart and soul into any gym class sport! (I still remember screaming and holding my gym suit together while I ran for the change room.)

Most women I know have a gym class horror story or two to share—stories that go a long way toward explaining why so many of us have grown up hating exercise. Take my friend Dawnette, for example. It was only after she became an adult that she managed to overcome her lifelong hatred for anything that even remotely resembled sports: "I used to hate to exercise," she admits. "I'm not athletic at all and I was teased about this a lot when I was growing up. As an adult, however, I've learned that there are ways to exercise as an individual that are more interesting and that I'm reasonably good at doing."

It's a shame that the one thing that our gym class teachers forgot to teach us was perhaps the most important lesson of all: moving your body can actually be fun!

The Best Excuses for Not Exercising

As if the horror of gym class weren't enough for us to contend with—and, frankly, you've got to wonder how many therapists have made their fortunes helping

---

The Skinny

"I think a lot of women hate exercising because they measure themselves against the TV commercials that show air-brushed, perky-breasted, super-thin women. They feel that there's just no way that they're ever going to look that way (which is true, because they aren't going to have their bodies airbrushed or their breasts enhanced via a computer!)"

— Amy, who is currently trying to lose weight

women to work through that particular trauma!—many of us spent our early adult years bouncing from aerobics class to aerobics class. (I suppose these aerobics classes were fun for the more coordinated members of the class. For me, they were an exercise in humiliation. Not only was I perpetually out of breath: I found it impossible to master all the fancy footwork that was inevitably required.) The end result of these less-than-positive experiences with exercise is that many of us have come up with a whole smorgasbord of reasons for hitting the couch instead of the gym! Here are just a few:

- **"Exercise is boring."** If your definition of exercising involves standing in the middle of your basement and skipping rope, you're right: it is boring. Fortunately, it doesn't have to be this way. There are plenty of ways to pump fun into any workout: go for a walk with a friend, watch TV while you ride your exercise bike, or wear your Walkman while you hit the Stairmaster at the gym. And if you're not up to that, walk around the perimeter of the grocery store once or twice before you do your shopping — or park a few blocks away from your bank when you hit the ATM.
- **"I'm just not the athletic type."** If at first you don't succeed, then hang up your running shoes for good, right? Wrong! Instead of throwing in the towel altogether, choose a less demanding activity. If you can't keep up with the aerobic class instructor's fancy footwork, go for a walk with a friend instead.
- **"I might get hurt."** You're right: there is some risk involved in biking or rollerblading on busy downtown streets. But there's an even greater risk to your health in not being active at all. If high-risk activities make your hair stand on end, then find a safer alternative. Whatever you do, don't bench yourself. Get back in the game.
- **"I'm too embarrassed to exercise."** If it's fear of looking foolish that's holding you back from getting active, relax. Contrary to what you might think, there are far more Mimis and Roseannes than Madonnas and Demis at your typical fitness facility. Besides, even the natural-born skinnies at the gym and the swimming pool are so busy focusing on their own workouts that they barely take notice of the other people around them. And as for those subhuman few who do get their jollies out of making snide remarks about fat people—well, let's just assume that they'll get their just desserts in the end when middle-aged spread sets in!
- **"I hate feeling sore afterwards."** While you might feel a few aches and pains when you first start to get active, these complaints should be fairly minor and relatively short-lived. There's no reason for you to push your

body to the point where you feel so stiff and sore that you can hardly move. Forget what Jane Fonda used to say about going for the burn. The "no pain, no gain" fitness philosophy went out of style about the same time as disco-wear.

- **"I'm too busy to exercise."** Are you tempted to skip your morning shower on a busy day? Probably not. That's because starting your day with a clean body is a priority to you. (Besides, it makes you a whole lot popular with those around you!) You need to give exercise the same priority in your schedule. In order to keep the exercise ball in the air, you have to be prepared to let a few other balls come tumbling down. Leave your bed unmade in the morning and let that last load of laundry go unfolded at night: those sacrifices are a small price to pay if it means that you can find 10 minutes at the start and end of each day to squeeze in a mini-workout. (Hint: Having to pull an unfolded bra out of the dryer in the morning won't kill you. Giving your heart muscle an extended vacation just might.)

- **"I can't afford to join a gym."** A gym membership can be a great motivator if you're serious about getting fit. Not only do you get inspired by seeing tons of other people working hard at getting fit: you're motivated to hit the gym yourself because you don't want to miss too many workouts when you're forking over $40 a month in membership fees! Still, you don't have to join a gym in order to be physically active. Think of all the fitness activities you can do for free (or almost free): walking around the block, exercising in front of the TV, strength-training in your kitchen while you're making dinner. The sky's the limit when it comes to finding budget-friendly ways to get fit.

- **"I'm too tired."** If you're feeling dragged out, you can't afford not to exercise. Contrary to popular belief, exercise helps to boost (not zap) your energy level. So if you're looking for a way to put a bit of bounce back into your step (or to keep your eyes open at your desk in the middle of the afternoon), hit the gym, not the coffee pot.

The Skinny

"When I first started going to the gym, I felt so out of place. I remember the first time I got weighed and I lost 7 pounds I was so excited! There was no one to tell, but I yelled it out anyway. A lady came running out of the change room to congratulate me. She said she had seen me on the treadmill and thought I was doing so well. I was floored. I thought people were looking at me and saying, 'Look at the fat girl.' Maybe some of them were, but this lady told me that she thought I was doing great. She congratulated me on the loss and told me to keep up the great work. I don't feel nearly so out of place now."

— Krista, who has lost more than 50 pounds over the past year

- **"I'm just not motivated enough to stick with a fitness program."** We all have days when we'd rather flake out on the couch than do as much as a single arm curl. Fortunately, there are plenty of ways to keep yourself motivated. If the idea of paying for that fitness club membership isn't enough to keep you motivated (and, frankly, it usually does the trick for me!), try coming up with other ways of keeping yourself all fired up about getting fit. Exercise with a friend, join a fitness class, give yourself a series of rewards for sticking with your fitness program (clothing in a smaller size is usually enough to get you hitting the Stairmaster with great enthusiasm!), and start keeping written records of your fitness progress so that you can celebrate your milestone achievements. (I still remember the first time I managed to run for 20 minutes on the treadmill at the gym. I was so pumped that I hopped off the machine and shared my news with the front desk staff! One of the people in the gym at the time was so happy for me that she sent me a card. It was waiting for me the next time I showed up to work out.)

What You Can Do to Turn Your Attitude Around

Having a love-hate relationship with exercise? (You love the idea of being fitter, but you hate the idea of actually working out!) Here are some steps you can take to turn your attitude around.

Stop Viewing Exercise as a Punishment

Here's one sure way to take the fun out of fitness: keep reminding yourself that it's something you have to do if you're really going to lose weight! "I think my problem is—and this is probably the case with a great number of women—that when you are exercising to lose weight, it becomes a chore rather than a fun activity," explains Heather, who has been struggling with her weight since she was a child. "It's no longer a case of saying to yourself, 'It's beautiful outside. I'm going to go walk on the beach and get some fresh air.' It becomes a case of, 'I'm fat and therefore I have to exercise.' It's like exercise is your punishment for being fat. You know that you are no longer walking for the fun of it, but for a reason—to lose weight."

It's not hard to see why that kind of attitude ends up dampening your enthusiasm for being active. It's not unlike the performance anxiety that can strike in the bedroom when you're consciously trying to get pregnant. (Think it's hard being a woman? Imagine what it's like being a guy at a time like that!)

Rather than treating exercise as something you have to do, try to convince yourself that it's something that you want to do. (You may have to lie a little at first, but, over time, you'll start believing yourself!)

The Skinny

"I have always hated exercise. It has always seemed to me to be too much work. It also takes a lot of time—going to the gym and then showering. Do I enjoy it now? You betcha! I feel such a sense of accomplishment when I finish either a TaeBo or Boxercise class at the gym. And I love getting in the hot sauna afterwards: it is like a reward for having succeeded in the workout."

— Krista, who has lost more than 50 pounds over the past year

Melissa was able to turn her negative attitude toward exercise on its head when she started focusing on the benefits of being active. Not only was she able to spend more time with her husband—he works out with her at the gym—she also had the opportunity to get to meet other women who were trying to improve their fitness level: "I get the chance to talk to other women who are in the same boat as me fitness-wise whenever I go to my water aerobics class."

Set Realistic Goals for Yourself

It's a fantasy that starts running through your head the moment you sign the membership contract at your local gym: within weeks—days even—you're going to see a remarkable change in your fitness level. Instead of huffing and puffing each time you have to lug a laundry basket upstairs, you're going to be taking the stairs two at a time. And instead of struggling to keep up with your two-year-old when he makes a breakaway at the park, you'll be tiring him out!

The problem with these fitness fantasies is that they end up setting you up for disappointment. As much as you might like to believe that a few hours on the treadmill is going to transform you into a Demi Moore, it's highly unlikely that your results are going to be quite that dramatic.

The Skinny

"Start slowly or you won't be able to stick to it. Don't work yourself too hard."

— Kathryn, who recently lost 70 pounds

A better approach is to set realistic fitness goals for yourself—goals that you have at least a fighting chance of achieving. Here are some things you may want to focus on:

- **The frequency of your workouts.** Promise yourself that you'll hit the gym or pound the pavement a certain number of times each week. Three times a week is generally considered to be the bare minimum, but one or two workouts is certainly better than none! Of course, you can certainly aim for more workouts than that if you're highly motivated. Just don't set yourself up for failure by promising yourself to exercise 366 days a year. (Hey, even the fitness clubs shut their doors at least one day of the year!)

- **The duration of your workouts.** Aim low rather than high until you really get into the swing of things. From a psychological standpoint at least, it's far better to aim to spend 20 minutes on the treadmill and achieve it than it is to set your sights on a 45-minute workout, but end up calling it quits in just half the time. (In the first scenario, you're left feeling like one of the runners in *Chariots of Fire*; in the second scenario, you're left feeling like an Olympic-calibre loser.)

- **The intensity of your workouts.** Do you want to burn 200 calories during that 20-minute workout, or would you be more than satisfied with kissing 100 calories goodbye? Be as specific as possible but, once again, don't aim for more than you can reasonably hope to achieve. Remember: you can always make your fitness goals more challenging as your fitness level improves.

Food for Thought

Sometimes it pays to think small. A recent study revealed that novice exercisers who initially commit to 10-minute exercise sessions are more likely to stick with their fitness programs than those who aim for lengthier workouts.

Sometimes it's fun to set little goals for yourself when you're in the middle of a workout—goals that you can achieve right then and there. "The other day when I was walking my dog, I tried to jog a bit," notes Margaret, who is currently exercising to lose weight. "I'm a terrible jogger, but I mentally set a goal for myself ('to the next corner') and tried to jog that far."

Choose an Activity That's Suited to Your Current Fitness Level

Does your vision of Hell include 24-hour-a-day aerobics classes led by a power-hungry masochist in thigh-high black boots? Then aerobics classes are probably not the ideal fitness activity for you. Rather than signing up for a high-intensity workout that you'll dread rather than enjoy, why not choose an exercise that's better suited to your current fitness level?

If you've been inactive for a considerable length of time, then walking is probably as good a place as any to start. You can gradually pick up the pace and increase the length of your walks as your fitness level improves. Then, if walking begins to lose its challenge, you can switch to an activity that's a little more demanding: jogging, biking, or perhaps even one of those dreaded aerobics classes!

Fortunately, there are lots of different activities to choose from. As you can see from Table 4.1, walking is the most popular fitness activity for Canadian women, but there are plenty of other great ways to stay active.

Here are some factors to consider when you're choosing a fitness activity:

- **Is it something that you will enjoy doing?** You have enough tasks to accomplish in a day. Don't make exercise one more "chore" to add to your to do list. Take the drudgery out of exercise by choosing activities that you will genuinely enjoy doing. For some women, that may be swimming. For others, skating. It doesn't matter what type of activity you choose as long as it's something you'll look forward to doing on a regular basis.
- **Is it something that you can fit into your schedule easily?** There's no point signing up for Saturday morning aerobics classes if they're likely to conflict with your son's hockey games. And there's no point in pretending you're going to drag your weary bones out of bed at 6:00 a.m. to make an early-morning fitness class at the gym if you're simply not a morning person. When you're choosing a fitness activity, try to find one that will fit your schedule easily. The more convenient it is for you to exercise, the more likely you are to actually do it.
- **Does it suit your "fitness personality"?** Group fitness activities like aerobics classes and group cycling classes are naturals for the extroverts of the world

The Skinny

"Exercise doesn't have to mean running a marathon every day. It can be a quick, easy twenty-minute walk around the block."

— Heather, who is currently trying to lose weight

Food for Thought

Here's a great excuse for passing on that group cycling class until your fitness level improves. The dropout rate for high-intensity fitness activities is twice as high as for moderate-intensity programs.

TABLE 4.1

THE TEN MOST POPULAR FITNESS ACTIVITIES FOR CANADIAN WOMEN

1. Walking	91%
2. Gardening and yard work	76%
3. Home exercise	57%
4. Swimming	54%
5. Social dancing	53%
6. Bicycling	41%
7. Bowling	29%
8. Exercise class/aerobics	28%
9. Skating	27%
10. Jogging/running and weight training	24%

Source: *Foundation for Joint Action: Reducing Physical Inactivity* by Cora Lynn Craig, Storm J. Russell, Christine Cameron, and Angele Beaulieu. Ottawa: Canadian Fitness and Lifestyle Research Institute, 1999.

(you know, the folks who clap their hands and cheer along with the aerobics instructor!), while solo activities like hitting the treadmill or the Stairmaster may be a better fit for the introverts of the world (those of us who prefer to wear our headphones and tune out everyone around us while we're working out). If you choose a fitness activity that suits your "fitness personality," you'll be more likely to stick with it.

- **Is the activity likely to aggravate any pre-existing injuries or medical conditions?** It's always a good idea to check with your doctor before starting a fitness program, but it's particularly important to do so if you've got any pre-existing health problems or chronic medical conditions. As a rule of thumb, you should plan to schedule a pre-workout checkup if you have a history of heart problems, chest pains, faintness, or dizzy spells; if you have high blood pressure; if you have a bone or joint problem, such as arthritis, that could be aggravated by the wrong types of exercise; if you're inactive and over the age of 65; if you are taking prescription medications; or you have other types of health problems that might limit your participation in physical activity. In most cases, your doctor will give you the go-ahead to proceed with your fitness program, but, in some cases, he or she may suggest that you stick to low-intensity workouts (e.g., walking) or workouts that are less likely to put any strain on your joints (e.g., swimming).

- **Can you afford any necessary equipment or membership fees?** Not all fitness activities were created equal—at least when it comes to the bottom line! If you're on a tight budget, you might want to forgo the membership at the local tennis club and sign up for a more budget-friendly water aerobics class at the local Y instead. Note: If you're thinking of joining a gym, make sure you find out about any hidden membership costs before you sign on the dotted line. While the federal government has forced most fitness clubs to clean up their act in recent years, some still resort to sleazy sales techniques in order to get you to purchase a fitness membership. (You can find out what to look for in a fitness club and what types of questions to ask by using the checklist in Table 4.2.)

TABLE 4.2

CHECKLIST FOR CHOOSING A FITNESS CLUB

Not sure what to look for in a fitness club? Here are some points to consider:

- How well do the centre's hours of operation fit your schedule?
- Is the fitness centre conveniently located?
- Is there free on-site parking available?
- Is there inexpensive on-site child-care available?
- Are the facilities clean and well-maintained?
- Is the equipment up-to-date and fully functional?
- Are there lineups for the types of equipment that you intend to use?
- Are there lineups for equipment at the times of the day when you are most likely to be using the centre?
- Is there enough equipment to allow you to switch to more challenging activities as your fitness level improves?
- Are there a variety of different types of fitness classes offered (e.g., both high-impact and low-impact classes)?
- Are any of the fitness classes offered designed to meet the needs of beginners?
- Do you feel comfortable at the centre?
- Are there other people your age and/or your size using the centre?
- Is the exercise area supervised by qualified instructors?
- Have centre staff members completed first aid and/or CPR training?
- Are the staff members who are responsible for conducting fitness appraisals properly trained and/or certified by an accredited fitness organization?
- Are the staff members experienced in developing fitness programs for women who have a significant amount of weight to lose?
- Are the staff members supportive of and respectful towards club members who have a significant amount of weight to lose?
- How long has the centre been in business?
- Does the centre have a good reputation in the community?
- Have any complaints against the centre been registered with any government departments or consumer watchdog organizations?
- What is the centre's philosophy?
- Does the centre offer a balanced approach to fitness and conditioning, or is the emphasis purely on weight loss?
- Is the fitness centre willing to allow you to try out their facilities for free before you sign on the dotted line?
- Do staff members receive any type of commission for recruiting new members?

Source: Adapted from a checklist in *The Body Image Directory: A Guide to Resources in Peterborough County*. Published by the Body Image Coalition, June 1996.

Start Slowly and Build on Your Successes

It's only natural to want to improve your fitness level overnight. (Frankly, I've always believed that this patience thing is highly overrated!) Unfortunately, it's not realistic to expect to be able to transform yourself from a couch potato to a marathon runner within days of starting your fitness program, nor is it healthy to attempt to do too much too soon.

Most of the women I know who've been able to make fitness a permanent part of their lives have started slowly and then built on their successes. This was certainly Kathryn's plan of attack—and one that paid off big-time for her: "I started by using workout videotapes at home—the most basic ones I could find, actually," she recalls. "I was really out of shape. I started by doing just a half hour of an aerobics video three days a week. Then I added more time to it and tried other tapes after about a month. Each month, I'd add on to this routine somehow, whether it was by increasing the time I spent during each session or by increasing the number of days I was working out each week. I would also set goals for myself, like, 'I'm going to work out four days this week.' I was pretty good about keeping my promises to myself, and I was careful not to push myself too hard or to set goals I couldn't meet."

Food for Thought

Here's some good news for you if you're more inclined to exercise at home than at the gym. A recent Stanford University study revealed that people who exercise in their own homes are more likely to stick with their fitness programs than people who work out elsewhere. What's more, a University of Florida study confirmed what many exercise physiologists have long suspected: people who exercise at home tend to lose more weight over the course of a year than people who exercise at other locations.

Inject Some Fun into Your Workouts

Who ever said that workouts have to be deadly boring or super serious? You're more likely to stay on track if your workouts are fun. Frankly, the sky's the limit when it comes to adding spice to your workout:

- **Change your routine.** Getting bored with your workout? Try something different for a change. Instead of hitting the treadmill each and every time you hit the gym, head for the exercise bikes or the Stairmaster instead. (Psst.....The technical term for using different pieces of equipment each time you work out is *cross-training*. If you drop that bit of lingo around the gym, you'll impress the heck out of all the jocks and jockettes you encounter. Just so you know, cross-training is considered to be a good thing: it allows you to work on a lot more muscle groups than you'd be able to work on if you stuck to a single piece of exercise equipment.) If you're running out of ideas on how to inject some fun into your workout, consider contracting the services of a personal trainer. For a one-time investment of $30 to $50 (the going rate for a one-hour fitness consultation), you could end up with an exciting new fitness program that's custom-designed to meet your own unique fitness needs.

The Skinny

"I change my exercise routine every two or three months. Right now I'm doing jogging and weight training. I'm getting ready to start learning tennis and I plan on taking an aerobics class in a few weeks."

— Kathryn, who has lost 70 pounds over the past year

- **Flip on some tunes.** Finding it hard to motivate yourself to run around the block? Grab your Walkman and your favourite music tape. There's something about exercising to music that almost makes you forget how hard you're working your body. (You'll note that I said "almost"!)

- **Exercise with a friend.** Misery loves company, right? (Hey, I'm only kidding!) Exercising with a friend could be the cure for even the worst case of the "I don't want to work out" blues! Kathryn is the first to admit that it's the opportunity to hang out with her buddy Karen that has her hitting the gym on a regular basis: "We watch *Jerry Springer*, gossip about people we know, and complain about our significant others!"

The Skinny

"If you're getting into a rut when it comes to doing your in-home aerobic workout, swap exercise videos with a friend or tape a bunch of TV exercise shows. Or use the 'picture-in-picture' feature on your TV set so that you can watch your favourite TV show and do your exercise tape at the same time!"

— Ann Douglas, *Sanity Savers: The Canadian Working Woman's Guide to Almost Having It All*

- **Hit the great outdoors.** If you're getting tired of working out in your basement or at the local gym, take your workout outdoors. Sometimes a change of scenery is all it takes to recharge your workout batteries. While our Canadian climate is less than ideal (how's that for understatement!), it's possible to exercise in both heat and cold if you follow some sensible precautions. (See Table 4.3.)

- **Don't forget to schedule some downtime.** Familiarity breeds contempt—especially where your workout's concerned. Some studies have shown that you don't achieve any marked improvement in your fitness level by exercising seven days a week as opposed to five days a week, so give your body a break and take some time off.

TABLE 4.3

TIPS ON EXERCISING IN EXTREMELY HOT OR COLD WEATHER

Don't be a fair-weather exerciser! Here are some tips on exercising in extremely hot or cold weather:

WHEN IT'S HOT OUTSIDE

- Plan your workout for the cooler and less humid times of day. Rather than exercising at high noon on the hottest day of the year, work out first thing in the morning or in the evening.
- Dress for success. Wear light-coloured, loose-fitting clothing to keep yourself as comfortable as possible while you're exercising.
- Drink plenty of fluids—but make sure they're the right type. If that ice-cold bottle of beer starts calling your name on a hot summer's day, plug your ears. Not only is beer packed with calories (a button-popping 12 calories per fluid ounce!) it also encourages dehydration—the last thing you need on a hot summer's day. Your best bets in the beverage department are water and specially formulated sports drinks such as Gatorade.
- Listen to your body. Stop exercising immediately if you experience muscle cramps or dizziness. You could be suffering from heat exhaustion.

WHEN IT'S COLD OUTSIDE

- Dress the part. Wear clothing that will keep you warm and dry while you're working out. High-tech fabrics such as polypropylene don't just look good, they're also designed to draw sweat away from the body and into the next layer of clothing—something that will help to keep you toasty warm.
- Learn to love the layered look. Dressing in layers isn't just trendy—it makes a lot of sense from a physiological standpoint. If you get overheated when you're exercising, you can peel off a layer or two. Start with a layer of polypropylene and then top it with a layer of fleece or wool to keep you warm. Then pop a lightweight polyester jacket on top of these two layers to protect yourself against the wind and rain.
- Don't forget your hands. Be sure to wear gloves or mitts to protect your hands from the harsh winter weather. (If you're smart, you'll make sure you're wearing a jacket with big pockets so that you can remove your gloves or mitts if your hands start to get too warm.)
- Put your best foot forward. Wear sensible footwear: warm, well-constructed boots with non-skid soles. The last thing you want to do is to put your workouts on ice because you've slipped and broken your arm!
- Top off your look with a great hat. It's common knowledge that you lose up to 40 percent of your body's heat through your neck and head. That's why it's important to keep both areas covered when you're exercising in the cold winter weather. You can either go with a hat and scarf or a balaclava (a particularly good bet if you suffer from breathing problems such as asthma, since the balaclava will help to warm your breath before it hits your lungs).
- Don't forget your water bottle. Believe it or not, you can get dehydrated in the winter months, too. If you're planning a lengthy workout, tote your water bottle along, too. (Note: This is particularly important if you're asthmatic, since people with respiratory disorders face a higher-than-average risk of becoming dehydrated during exercise.)
- Watch for signs of hypothermia. If you start experiencing shivering, drowsiness, or disorientation, it's time to put the brakes on your workout.

Make Fitness a Priority in Your Life

Finding it hard to find the time to exercise? You're certainly in good company—57% of the women surveyed by the Melpomene Institute (a U.S. women's health research organization) reported that work pressures kept them from being active, while another 39.4% blamed family commitments for keeping them from exercising on a regular basis.

There's no denying it: most of us do have too many balls in the air. What we need to do, however, is to make sure that exercise is one of the balls that stays airborne! While we women are pros when it comes to putting everyone else's needs ahead of our own, exercise is one area in which we owe it to ourselves—and those who love us—to be a little selfish. We need to remind ourselves that we aren't going to do anyone any good—ourselves included!—if we skip our workouts on a regular basis.

"You have to make exercise part of your day and set aside some time for it," says Heather, a recent fitness convert. "You would never say you don't have time to shower: you have to give exercise the same amount of priority."

Here are some tips on fitting exercise into even the most insanely busy schedule:

- Commit to exercising on a regular basis. "Make exercise a priority," suggests Amy, who has been exercising in an effort to lose weight. "Treat it like a meeting that you can't get out of."
- Focus on mini-workouts. If you can't find the time to squeeze a full-length workout into your day, try fitting in a couple of 10-minute mini-workouts instead. A recent study at the Brown University School of Medicine and the University of Pittsburgh revealed that short bouts of exercise sprinkled throughout the day are every bit as effective as longer bouts of exercise performed all at once. (Note: You can find a smorgasbord of suggestions about ways to fit exercise into your day in Table 4.4.)
- Exercise with a friend or family member. Rather than visiting over a cup of coffee, go for a walk or a bike ride instead. Better yet, sign up for water aerobics classes or join a baseball team together—

The Skinny

"Exercising was my biggest challenge because I strongly disliked it. I had real trouble getting motivated to work out, particularly in the beginning when I had no positive feedback or visible results to encourage me. In order to make myself exercise, I set mental goals for myself, like telling myself that I'm going to work out three days this week no matter what. I try to set realistic goals so that I won't get discouraged or have trouble achieving them."

— Kathryn, who has lost 70 pounds over the past year

The Skinny

"I keep a small weight by the computer and use it when I have time. I walk whenever I can. I use stairs instead of elevators. I try to make anything I can into an exercise. I'll do leg lifts when I'm reading or washing dishes, for example."

— Catherine, who has lost 15 pounds

The Skinny

that way, you'll be committed to exercising together on a regular basis.

- Make it easy for yourself to exercise. Keep a fully packed gym bag by the front door. That way, you won't have to waste half your workout time trying to track down a pair of running shoes—or, even worse, arrive at the gym only to discover that you haven't got anything to wear on the treadmill but a pair of winter boots. (Been there, done that, don't want to do it again!)

- Double up on other tasks so that you can "buy" yourself more time to exercise. We women are famous for multi-tasking. The problem is that we sometimes forget to set aside the extra time that we've "bought" ourselves by doing two or more things at once. So next time you spend an hour making a spaghetti dinner for the freezer and a chicken stir-fry for tonight's dinner at the same time, make a mental note that you've just bought yourself an hour of exercise time.

- Let others in your life know that fitness has become a priority for you. They may be willing to pick up some of the slack around the house if that makes it easier for you to get to the gym. If they're not willing to pitch in and help, don't be afraid to look outside the family to get the help you need. Hire a teenager to come over and fold a couple of loads of laundry so that you'll have time to go for a walk with a friend.

TABLE 4.4

20 RELATIVELY PAIN-FREE WAYS TO SQUEEZE EXERCISE INTO YOUR DAY

1. Do a set of abdominal crunches before you hop out of bed in the morning.
2. Hop on your exercise bike while your kids are eating breakfast.
3. Work some stretching into your morning shower routine.
4. Ride your bike to work.
5. Take the stairs rather than the elevator when you arrive at the office. (A Yale University study revealed that only 5% of Americans—and just 1% of overweight Americans—take the stairs when both the stairs and an elevator are available. Frankly, I think we'd be kidding ourselves if we tried to pretend that we Canadians are a superior breed.)
6. Take a quick walk during your lunch hour. You'll clear your head and burn off calories at the same time.
7. Hit the gym on your way home from work. If you go straight home, you might be reluctant to head back out again after dinner.

8. Do some abdominal crunches when you're waiting for the pasta to finish cooking. (Hey, what else are you going to do with that eight- to ten-minute chunk of time?)

9. Reach for your free weights if the folks at Revenue Canada put you on hold. Just remember to put the weights down gently when they tell you the bad news about your tax return.

10. Keep canned goods and other essentials in the basement so you'll have an excuse for running up and down stairs more often.

11. Play with your kids. Use your infant or toddler as a free weight while you're playing on the floor or play tag with your preschooler or school-aged child.

12. Pop an exercise tape into the VCR and convince your kids to do the workout with you. They'll find it hilariously funny, and you'll likely manage to squeeze in a few leg lifts in between giggles.

13. Sign your kids up for swimming lessons and take a water fitness class yourself at the same time. It's a hassle-free way to solve at least one of your scheduling nightmares.

14. Toss your baby in the stroller and run around the block. (You might want to pick up one of those super-durable jogging strollers if you intend to do this manoeuvre on a regular basis.)

15. Turn laundry folding into a form of interval training. Fold ten garments and then run them upstairs. Fold another ten garments and then run them upstairs. Repeat until you run out of laundry, time, or energy!

16. Keep a set of dumbbells in your bathroom cupboard so that you can squeeze in a few arm curls while you're watching your toddler play in the tub.

17. Ditch some of the labour-saving devices in your home. You'll burn plenty of extra calories over the course of a year by retiring the TV remote and the automatic garage door opener.

18. Don't use the moving sidewalks at the airport. Seize the opportunity to stretch your legs before you end up being strapped into an airplane seat for a couple of hours.

19. Get off the bus a block or two early or park your car a block or two further away when you're running errands. It's an easy way to force yourself to squeeze a few extra minutes of walking into your day.

20. If your doctor or dentist is running behind schedule, go for a short walk rather than sitting there fidgeting in the waiting room.

Stick with Your Workout Long Enough to Start Reaping the Benefits

Don't get discouraged with your apparent lack of progress if you don't develop buns of steel within the first couple of weeks of hitting the gym. It takes time to burn off fat and to build up muscle tissue. If you throw in the towel too soon, you'll end up cheating yourself of the potential benefits of becoming fit.

Consider what Amy—a true fitness aficionado—has to say about the matter: "I think a lot of women hate exercise because they don't really give it a chance. I don't know very many people who have tried aerobics or some other activity and stuck with it for two or three weeks who don't end up loving it. It's a thrilling experience to see your body expand its capabilities and

The Skinny

"I pick up my weights when I am watching TV. Those two to three minutes of commercials are a great time to work in a weight-lifting exercise or even a floor exercise or two."

—Tammy, who is currently trying to shed two babies' worth of "baby fat"

The Skinny

"If it's hard at first, hang in there: it will get easier. Your body just needs to adjust."

— Heather, who recently started exercising in order to lose weight

to push yourself to new limits. I think many women don't realize how thrilling it is until they give it a try."

Kathryn—who recently discovered the joys of working out for herself—agrees: "I absolutely love exercise now. I think what really helped me enjoy it was getting out of the house. I don't use workout tapes at all anymore, although they were a real saving grace when I first started out. I like taking aerobics classes and I enjoy working out with my exercise buddy, Karen. I also enjoy the challenge of my gym workouts because I feel strong while I'm doing them. I can feel and see the results. That probably makes a big difference."

If you're having a particularly miserable time working out—you have nightmares about the Stairmaster before you hit the gym or you start cursing the aerobics instructor the moment she bounces into the room—perhaps it's time to consider switching to another type of fitness activity. Don't beat yourself up for making a poor choice in fitness activities the first time around, even if your mistake ends up costing you a bit of money: just chalk it off as a bad date gone wrong and start looking for the workout of your dreams again.

What Exercise Can Do for Your Weight-Loss Program

If I offered to sell you a magic potion that would burn calories, boost your metabolic rate, help to reduce your appetite, and increase your feeling of well-being, you'd have your credit card out in a flash.

Believe it or not, exercise can deliver all of these benefits and a whole lot more. Consider the facts for yourself:

- **Exercise helps your body to burn calories.** Your body needs fuel in order to move. It gets this fuel from the food that you have just eaten and/or the fat that your body previously stashed away for just such a rainy day. The more vigorously you exercise, the more calories your body burns. (See Table 4.5.)

TABLE 4.5

THE NUMBER OF CALORIES PEOPLE OF VARIOUS WEIGHTS BURN THROUGH VARIOUS TYPES OF EXERCISE

ACTIVITY (20 MINUTES)	BODY WEIGHT		
	125 pounds	175 pounds	250 pounds
Cycling at 5.5 mph	84	116	166
Cycling at 13 mph	178	248	356
Dancing	96	132	188
Golf	66	96	136
Racquetball	150	208	288
Running at 5.5 mph	180	250	356
Running at 7 mph	236	328	464
Skiing, cross country	188	276	388
Skiing, downhill	160	224	320
Skiing, water	120	176	260
Squash	150	208	288
Swimming (front crawl)	80	112	160
Tennis	112	160	230
Walking at 2 mph	58	80	116
Walking at 4 mph	104	144	204

Source: Adapted from a similar table in *Thin for Life* by Anne Fletcher. Shelburne, Vermont: Chapters Publishing, 1994.

- **Exercise boosts your metabolic rate during and immediately after your workout.** Your body doesn't just burn more calories while you're exercising. It continues to burn more calories at a higher-than-normal rate for about an hour after each workout (or for as long as 12 hours after your workout, if you're a highly trained athlete).

- **Exercise helps you to build muscle tissue.** Since muscle tissue burns more calories than fat tissue, your body will burn more calories as you build up muscle tissue. This can help to offset the drop in metabolism that typically occurs when you go on a diet (see Chapter 2, "The Dirt on Diets.") The results can be surprisingly dramatic: one Tufts University study showed that people who increased their muscle mass by just 3 pounds over a 12 week period could eat 15% more calories without gaining weight.

The Skinny

Here's some good news for you if you're toting around a few extra pounds: the heavier you are, the more calories you burn when you exercise. While a 125-pound woman can expect to burn off about 80 calories during a 20 minute swim, a 250-pound woman will burn twice as many calories during the same workout.

Food for Thought

Men are more likely to experience a decrease in appetite after working out than women.

- **Exercise can help to curb your appetite.** Your appetite tends to decrease when you're exercising—something that can make it easier for you to lose weight. There's just one bit of fine print you need to know about: while your appetite is likely to decrease after moderate exercise, it can go through the roof after a bout of vigorous exercise. The moral of the story? Don't overdo it at the gym.

- **Exercise can increase your overall sense of well-being.** That can make it easier for you to stick with your weight-loss program. After all, you're less likely to hit the vending machine if you're experiencing a "runner's high" from your workout.

- **Exercise can help you stay focused on your weight-loss goals.** "Exercise helps to keep my motivation high," explains Jill, who is halfway toward her goal of losing 120 pounds. "After all, I wouldn't dream of having pizza or some decadent dessert right after working out! What a waste that would be!"

- **Exercise can help you to maintain your weight loss once you reach your goal.** A recent study conducted at the Kaiser Permanente Medical Center in Fremont, California, revealed that 90% of the women who successfully maintained their weight loss exercised at least three times per week for 30 minutes or more.

The Skinny

"Exercise was the key to my losing weight. Becoming physically active was not just the boost my metabolism needed to help me shed the extra weight: it also provided me with the mindset I needed in order to be successful. Exercise made me feel strong and that feeling of strength translated into better willpower during the difficult periods."

— Jenna, who has lost 90 pounds over the past year

What Exercise Can Do for Your Overall Health

Losing weight isn't the only perk that goes along with becoming physically fit. Far from it! In fact, it's hard to imagine any other single change that you could make to your lifestyle that would result in such a big payoff in terms of your health. Consider the facts for yourself:

- **Exercise reduces your risk of developing heart disease.** It strengthens your heart muscle. It improves the flow of blood, oxygen, and nutrients to all muscles, including your heart. It brings both your systolic and diastolic blood pressure down by about 10 points. And it reduces the levels of "bad" cholesterol in your blood while boosting the levels of "good" cholesterol. (One study at Texas A & M University revealed that these blood cholesterol benefits can be enjoyed after a moderate-intensity workout on a stationary bike, a workout that's vigorous enough to burn about 350 calories, and that these effects typically last for 24 to 48 hours.)

- **Exercise reduces your chances of developing breast cancer.** Studies have shown that physically active women are 20 to 42 percent less likely to get breast cancer than sedentary women. Researchers believe that this decreased risk is due to a reduction in two key breast cancer risk factors: body weight and estrogen levels. (Women who are overweight tend to have higher levels of estrogen, and high levels of estrogen are known to play a role in breast cancer.)
- **Exercise reduces your chances of developing colon cancer.** People who exercise regularly are 60 percent less likely to develop colon cancer. This may be because exercise stimulates the intestinal muscles to excrete waste products more quickly, thereby minimizing the amount of time that cancer-causing substances in waste products come into contact with the colon.
- **Exercise reduces your chances of developing adult-onset diabetes.** It helps to remove some of the glucose from your blood by drawing upon this as a source of energy both during and after exercise.
- **Exercise reduces your chances of developing osteoporosis.** One U.S. government study of 238 post-menopausal women revealed that those who regularly walked a mile a day had denser bones and a slower rate of bone loss than women the same age who were less active.
- **Exercise improves your aerobic capacity.** It helps to increase the amount of oxygen your lungs use — something that's good for your entire body!
- **Exercise gives your immune system a boost.** Aerobic exercise helps to improve your immune system's ability to recognize such foreign invaders as bacteria and viruses. There's just a bit of fine print you need to know about: while exercise sessions of 30 to 60 minutes do good things for your immune system, after 90 minutes of strenuous exercise, your body starts releasing stress hormones that actually increase your odds of getting sick. The moral of the story? You *can* get too much of a good thing.

- **Exercise helps to counter the effects of osteoarthritis.** A study at the Maryland School of Medicine demonstrated that exercise combined with dietary changes can allow women with chronic knee pain to enjoy reduced pain and increased movement.
- **Exercise may help to reduce your risk of developing Alzheimer's disease.** A study at Care Western Reserve University revealed that people who exercise regularly between the ages of 20 and 59 are less likely to develop Alzheimer's disease after age 60.
- **Exercise is a highly effective relaxant.** One study found that a simple walk can decrease tension as much as a tranquilizer.
- **Exercise can help to improve your mood.** Researchers at Indiana University in Bloomington discovered that anxiety levels tend to dip for at least two hours after a workout.
- **Exercise helps to improve mental alertness.** A study at Middlesex University in the U.K. revealed that exercise can even make you more creative.
- **Exercise gives you an energy boost that lasts long after your workout is over.** It also helps to ensure that you get a good night's sleep—good news for anyone who suffers from insomnia.
- **Exercise improves your posture and balance.** That can improve your self-confidence and help to reduce back pain.
- **Exercise can boost your life expectancy.** One Harvard University study showed that graduates of the university who burned more than 1500 calories per week through exercise outlived their more sedentary classmates by two years.

Designing the Ultimate Workout

Now that we've talked about the benefits of physical activity, let's get down to the real nitty-gritty: what the experts recommend when it comes to designing a workout.

There are three main ingredients in the recipe for the ultimate workout: endurance training (sometimes referred to as the aerobic or cardiovascular element of a workout), strength training, and flexibility training (also known as stretching).

Endurance Training

The term *endurance training* is used to describe those fitness activities that are designed to increase the endurance of your heart, lungs, and circulatory system. These are also the types of activities that tend to give you an energy boost—walking, jogging, running, cycling, skating, swimming, dancing, and so on.

The experts recommend that you do some endurance training four to seven days each week. Ideally, you should start with less intensive activities like walking, gradually increasing the intensity and duration of your workouts as you get more fit.

One of the biggest questions that beginners have about endurance training is how hard they should be working. There are two basic ways to measure the amount of effort that's going into your workout: by checking your pulse (see Table 4.6) and by assessing your rate of perceived exertion (see Table 4.7).

Food for Thought

Don't expect to burn off a lot of calories in the bedroom—unless, of course, that's where you keep your exercise bike. You only burn about 4.5 calories a minute during a typical romantic interlude.

TABLE 4.6

GET IN THE ZONE

To achieve maximum benefits from exercise, you should aim to get your heart rate into the aerobic zone. Your target heart rate zone is 50 to 75 percent of your maximum heart rate (the fastest your heart can beat). While you can get a more precise reading by considering your own resting heart rate, this table should give you a rough idea of how many times per minute your heart should be beating when you're doing endurance training.

AGE	TARGET HEART RATE ZONE (50 TO 75%)	AVERAGE MAXIMUM HEART RATE (100%)
20 to 30 years of age	98 to 146 beats per minute	195 beats per minute
31 to 40 years of age	93 to 138 beats per minute	185 beats per minute
41 to 50 years of age	88 to 131 beats per minute	175 beats per minute
51 to 60 years of age	83 to 123 beats per minute	165 beats per minute
61 years of age and older	78 to 116 beats per minute	155 beats per minute

Source: Weight-Control Information Network

Strength Training

Strength training involves using resistance (either the weight of your own body or a set of weights) to increase your strength. It helps your bones and muscles to stay strong, thereby improving your posture and helping to prevent diseases such as osteoporosis.

TABLE 4.7

MEASURING YOUR RATE OF PERCEIVED EXERTION (RPE)

The rate of perceived exertion scale (RPE) allows you to gauge the intensity of your workout by assessing how hard you feel you are working.

NUMERICAL RATING FOR THE WORKOUT	HOW YOU MIGHT DESCRIBE THE WORKOUT IN WORDS	TYPICAL ACTIVITIES
0	Resting	Watching TV or reading a book
1	Very light	Folding laundry
2	Light	Taking a leisurely stroll
3	Light	Walking slowly
4	Light/moderate	Doing light housework
5	Moderate	Walking at a moderate pace or working in your garden
6	Moderate/hard	Walking at a fast pace
7	Hard	Jogging briskly or cycling up and down hills
8	Very hard	Working hard on the Stairmaster or crosstrainer at the gym
9	Very hard/extremely hard	Sprinting on a flat surface
10	Extremely hard	Sprinting up a steep hill

Source: Adapted from *Fitness for Dummies* by Suzanne Schlosberg and Liz Neporent. Chicago, IL: IDG Books, 1996

The experts recommend that you include strength training in your workout two to four days each week. To reduce the risk of injury, you should get in the habit of starting your strength-training session with five minutes of endurance training and flexibility training. Once you've warmed up, you can then proceed to do two to four sets of ten to fifteen repetitions each of a variety of different exercises: overhead presses, arm curls, hamstring stretches, and so on. You can either ask the fitness instructor at the gym to design a strength-training program for you or you can use an off-the-shelf program, such as the one outlined in *Strong Women Stay Slim* by Miriam E. Nelson and Sarah Wernick—the program I use, incidentally.

Here are some important points to keep in mind if you're new to the world of strength training:

- You need to ensure that your strength-training program covers all of the major muscle groups—your arms, your torso, and your legs—and that you make a point of working both sides of your body as well as sets of opposing muscles. Not only

Food for Thought

"Muscles are beautiful. Strength is beautiful. Muscle tissue is beautiful. It is metabolically, medically, and philosophically beautiful."

— Natalie Angier, *Woman: An Intimate Geography*

will you end up with a more symmetrical body; you'll reduce your chance of injury.

- Make sure that you've got your technique down pat. Proper training is important if you want to protect your back and joints from undue stress.
- Be sure to breathe while you're lifting. (You'll instinctively want to hold your breath.)
- Make sure that you take at least one day off in between strength-training sessions. Your muscles need time to recover from the previous session.

Flexibility Training

Go figure: despite overwhelming evidence about its benefits, flexibility training continues to be the Rodney Dangerfield of the exercise world—a key element of fitness that doesn't get nearly the respect it deserves. While many of us pay lip service to the importance of stretching, very few of us actually follow through.

Flexibility training can help to improve your overall quality of life. It prevents your muscles from losing their flexibility, something that can eventually make it more difficult for you to carry out your everyday activities and that puts you at greater risk of experiencing falls, sprained muscles, and other injuries.

The experts recommend that you include flexibility training in your workout four to seven days per week. As a rule of thumb, you should plan to spend as much time on stretching as you do on the other elements of your fitness routine. In other words, if you're spending 20 minutes on endurance training and 20 minutes on strength training, you should plan to squeeze in 20 minutes of flexibility training as well.

In addition to formal stretching programs (once again, you'll find plenty of suggested exercises in the growing number of books that focus on the art of stretching), there are a number of other activities that can help to improve your flexibility: gardening, yard work, golf, bowling, yoga, curling, dance, and even vacuuming. (Don't worry: that last one is our little secret!)

Fat Chance

Before you get carried away and start fantasizing about getting as lean-and-mean as Arnold Schwarzenegger, put down your dumbbells and give yourself a quick reality check. Because men are designed to have more lean body mass than women, their percentage of body fat is considerably lower. While anything over 27% to 30% percent body fat is considered too much for a woman, a man is labelled overweight the moment his body-fat percentage passes the 23% to 25% percent mark. (Similarly, a woman is labelled obese once her body fat percentage exceeds 32%, while a man is labelled obese as soon as he reaches 28%.)

The Skinny

Work stretching into your daily routine. Don't reserve stretching for the gym. Do it in the morning while you're in the shower, in the daytime when you're working at your computer, and in the evening when you're watching TV.

To maximize the effectiveness of stretching and minimize the risk of injury, it's important to pay careful attention to these six basic rules of stretching:

1. Warm up for a few minutes before you start stretching. It's easier and safer to stretch a warm muscle than a cold one. And don't forget to stretch after a workout: it helps to reduce any muscle aches you might experience the next day.
2. Be gentle. Forget what Jane Fonda said about going for the burn. Move into the stretch slowly and gradually until you feel tension in the muscle and connective tissue. If there's any pain, stop.
3. Hold each stretch for 30 seconds. Anything less than 30 seconds is ineffective.
4. Don't hold your breath during a stretch. Breathe normally and relax as completely as you can.
5. Don't bounce. While ballistic stretching (performing bouncing, repetitive motions while stretching) may be the latest fad, most experts advise against the practice. Abrupt bouncing motions cause the muscles to contract rather than stretch.
6. Stretch both sides. Always stretch the left and the right (or the front and the back) of an area. This will allow you to maintain balance and symmetry—something that helps to enhance flexibility and performance while reducing the risk of injury.

Now that I've armed you with the facts about both healthy eating and exercise, it's time to move on and talk about another important ingredient in the recipe for weight-loss success: getting psyched up to make all these lifestyle changes!

5

Head Games

While it's tempting to look for shortcuts to the whole weight loss thing—to pass on the healthy dinner and the workout and hope instead that the Weight Loss Fairy will show up with her liposuction machine and zap those unwanted inches from your hips and thighs while you're sleeping!—you know in your heart that you can't expect to lose weight without making the types of lifestyle changes that we've been talking about over the past few chapters.

Unfortunately, as you've no doubt discovered by now, it's one thing to know what needs to be done and quite another to actually do it. In this chapter, we're going to consider ways that you can move beyond paying mere lip service to the idea of losing weight and actually start walking the talk. The first thing we're going to look at is how you go about determining whether or not you're actually ready to lose weight. (Believe it or not, you might be a bit more attached to that padding on your thighs than you're prepared to admit to yourself or anyone else!) Then we're going to don our lab coats and put the eating and exercise habits of those strange and exotic creatures known as naturally skinny women under the microscope.

The Skinny

"I spent some time mentally preparing myself to lose weight this time—or rather trying to calm myself down about the prospect of losing weight. I feel like losing weight is so over-whelming and impossible that I get myself all worked up over the prospect of trying to lose weight again. I've spent some time for the past month or so trying to 'talk' myself through it—trying to make myself shift the focus away from dieting and on to healthy eating. I think it might be working."

— Heather, who has just started trying to lose weight

Are You Ready to Take the Plunge?

It's one thing to flirt with the idea of losing weight; it's quite another to be prepared to make a commitment. Here are some points to consider when trying to decide whether you're ready to get involved with a weight-loss program.

How Long Have You Been Thinking About Losing Weight?

If your desire to lose weight is pretty much a spur-of-the-moment thing (the result of trying to slip into a pair of jeans that will no longer zip up or your reaction to some relative's less-than-tactful remark about the size of your behind), you may not be ready to embark on your weight-loss journey quite yet, girl-friend. As eager as you may be to hop that train to Slimsville, your trip will be pretty short if you're not psychologically ready to make the journey.

You see, as much as you might like to get rid of your weight woes quicker than you can say "cellulite," there's no express line to permanent weight loss. In fact, psychologists believe that you have to pass through five distinct stages if you're going to make lasting changes to your eating and exercise habits: precontemplation, contemplation, preparation, action, and mainte-nance (see Table 5.1). They argue that if you attempt to fast-forward through

TABLE 5.1

THE FIVE STAGES OF CHANGE

STAGE	HOW IT RELATES TO WEIGHT LOSS
Stage 1: Precontemplation	You're not even thinking about making changes to your eating or exercise habits.
Stage 2: Contemplation	You're flirting with the idea of changing your eating and exercise habits, but you haven't taken any concrete action yet.
Stage 3: Preparation	You've started to lay the groundwork for any changes you hope to make.
Stage 4: Action	You've started to make some changes to your eating and/or exer-cise habits.
Stage 5: Maintenance	You're comfortable with the changes you've made and you intend to stick with them.

these stages, you'll simply end up short-circuiting your weight-loss efforts.

If losing weight is something that you've been thinking about for a very long time and you've started to lay some of the necessary groundwork (e.g., you've joined a gym and you've started reading up on healthy eating), then you're probably ready to start making some changes. If, however, your decision to lose weight is a relatively spur-of-the-moment thing—the direct result of a bad experience with a tight pair of jeans or a less-than-tactful relative—perhaps you're not ready to hop that train to Slimsville quite yet. (As much as you might like to believe in quick fixes and miracle cures, I've got some bad news for you, Virginia: there isn't any Weight Loss Fairy!)

Food for Thought

Don't think of weight loss as an all-or-nothing proposition. Recent studies have shown that even a modest weight loss can deliver health benefits. In fact, one study reported in the *Journal of the American Medical Association* revealed that women who lost as little as five pounds handled everyday activities with greater ease and experienced fewer aches and pains.

Are You More Motivated Today than You've Been in the Past?

While there's no such thing as "the perfect time" to lose weight (remember, I broke that news to you back in Chapter 1!), people who have successfully lost weight and maintained their weight loss typically report that something "clicked" for them during their most recent attempt to lose weight.

"People who've lost weight and kept it off will tell you that the last time—the time that worked—they were 'finally ready'," notes Janis Jibrin in *The Unofficial Guide to Dieting Safely*. "They say that they were only 'kinda ready' during all the previous attempts, when they lost weight but gained it back. These earlier experiences taught them things that worked, and these they plugged into their lifestyles when they finally did get the proper motivation."

Have You Thought About Why You Want to Lose Weight?

The surest way to sabotage your weight-loss efforts is to attempt to lose weight for the wrong reasons. Trying to lose weight to impress a guy? You might was well order that truckload of M & Ms right now. (Hey, there's no point in postponing the inevitable!) The same goes for losing weight to please your parents, your kids, your best friend, or your boss. There's one good reason and one good reason only for attempting to lose weight: for yourself. Accept no substitutes!

Have You Thought About What Your Life Will Be Like After You Lose Weight?

If you're still harbouring some secret fantasy about how perfect your life will be when you finally lose weight, it's time to lose the fantasy, not the weight! While losing weight is never easy, women who have realistic ideas about what their life will be like when they lose weight are in for a far smoother ride than those who expect their weight loss to eliminate all of their problems. (Remember, we're talking about a weight-loss program here, not a magic wand!)

Have You Figured Out Why Your Past Attempts at Losing Weight Have Failed?

Here's some good news for you if your past attempts at losing weight have been less than successful: you can rely on what you've learned from those experiences to bolster your current weight-loss efforts. (Just think of it as a rather prolonged type of do-it-yourself consulting!)

Fell off the wagon last time because your program was too rigid? You can make sure that your current program is a whole lot more flexible.

Didn't have enough support from friends and family members the last time around? You can line up an entire cheerleading squad to cheer you on this time!

Just think of all those past attempts at weight loss as laying the groundwork for your current success. As Anne Fletcher notes in *Thin for Life*, "No matter what you weigh, how many times you've lost and regained weight, you are more knowledgeable now than you were before each weight-loss effort of the past."

Do You Have Time to Make These Types of Lifestyle Changes?

It takes time to hit the gym and prepare healthy meals for yourself. There's no doubt that this is a good use of your time—after all, what could be better than investing in your own health?—but it still takes time to make these types of lifestyle changes. Heck, even Oprah finds it hard to squeeze her workouts in—and she's got both a live-in chef and a personal trainer!

Have You Learned to Accept Your Body, for Better and for Worse?

You'd think that hating your body would be a guaranteed ticket to weight-loss success—that the thought of seeing yourself naked in the mirror would have you running into the arms of Jenny Craig.

Unfortunately, quite the opposite is true. The worse you feel about your body, the more likely your weight-loss efforts are to fail. Researchers at the

Stanford University School of Medicine have discovered that you're actually twice as likely to be successful at losing weight if you feel reasonably good about your body. (That means accepting your body, flaws and all, rather than groaning in dismay each time you catch a glimpse of your reflection in the mirror!)

Not exactly in love with your body? Don't panic. There's plenty you can do to turn your attitude around. Here are a few ideas to get you started:

The Skinny

"A little selfishness may be in order to achieve a healthier lifestyle. Other people in your family may have to work around your schedule for a change."

— Laura Fraser, *Losing It: False Hopes and Fat Profits in the Diet Industry*

- Think about the things that you like about your body rather than the things you don't like. Less than thrilled with the size of your hips? Don't give them a second thought. Instead, focus your energies on those parts of your body that you like the most.
- Consider what your body is capable of doing rather than what it looks like. Your body is a truly miraculous machine, capable of a performing a range of tasks that no computer could ever hope to carry out. Rather than getting hung up on the fact that you've got a few stretch marks on your abdomen or that you're carrying around some extra weight from your last pregnancy, why not choose instead to celebrate all the wonderful things that your body can do—not the least of which is giving birth to another human being!
- Remind yourself that perfect bodies only exist in Hollywood—and sometimes not even there. Did you know, for example, that the producers of *Pretty Woman* had to hire a body double to do the opening scenes of the movie because Julia Roberts's body wasn't quite perfect enough? Kind of helps to put things in perspective, now doesn't it?
- Be your own best friend. You'd never dream of telling your best friend that her hips were getting huge or that a particular skirt made her look fat and ugly. (If you did, she would no longer be your best friend!) Why not cut yourself the same slack?

Are You Creative When It Comes to Solving Problems?

One of the keys to permanent weight loss is being able to come up with creative solutions to situations which have traditionally caused a problem. "People who succeed at weight loss are confronted with the same high-risk situations as their diet-challenged cohorts," notes dietitian Elizabeth Somer in a recent article in *Shape* magazine. "The difference is that diet failures fall victim to these situations, while successes use creative problem solving."

Food for Thought

Are you guilty of substituting food for sleep? Studies have shown that sleep-deprived people tend to eat 10 to 15 percent more calories than people who are getting the rest they need. While it's tempting to turn to food when you need a quick pick-me-up, a better solution is to give your body what it really needs: a good night's sleep.

People who know how to think outside the box (particularly the Oreo cookie box!) are often able to sidestep weight-loss-related problems before they even occur. Someone who knows that she's going to finish off the rest of the cheesecake the moment her dinner guests leave can avoid the temptation entirely by sending the leftovers home with them.

Are You Ready to Change Your Attitudes Toward Food and Exercise—Not Just Your Behaviour?

Don't ever want to go on another "diet" again? I can't say I blame you. I mean, who would willingly sign up for the opportunity to starve themselves for a week or two and then gain all the weight they've lost back during a brief indiscretion with a box of Timbits?

If you're looking for the permanent solution to your weight problems—and, frankly, you'd be crazy to settle for anything but—you need to be prepared to change your attitudes toward food and exercise, not just your behaviour. That means designing a program that you can stick with over the long-run rather than some band-aid solution that won't last any longer than a couple of weeks. It's honesty time, girlfriend. Are you prepared to make this type of commitment?

Are You Ready to Do Battle with Emotional Eating?

Are you an emotional eater—someone who eats for emotional rather than physical reasons? If you're waving your hand frantically and vigorously nodding yes, you're certainly in good company. Emotional eating is a problem for a great many people, but tends to be a particular problem for women.

You can assume that emotional eating is a problem for you if you exhibit the following classic emotional eating behaviours:

- You are in the habit of eating when you're not hungry.
- You tend to lose control when you're eating certain foods (your so-called "trigger foods"), eating far more of them than your body necessarily wants or needs.
- You always eat everything on your plate—even if you're feeling stuffed halfway through your dinner.
- You head for the refrigerator or the vending machine as a means of avoiding an unpleasant task or confrontation.

- You use food as a sedative when you're feeling stressed, angry, lonely, or tired.
- You turn to food instead of taking care of your needs in other ways: finding time to relax, getting the sleep you need, and so on. ("Eating can become a quick way to try to do something nice for yourself when you don't have the time to really take care of yourself," writes Laura Fraser in *Losing It: False Hopes and Fat Profits in the Diet Industry*.)
- You eat more when you're alone than when you're with a group and you are in the habit of stashing away candy and other "forbidden foods" so that you can enjoy them in secret later on.
- You feel guilty or angry with yourself when you break down and eat foods that you think you shouldn't be eating.

The best way to pinpoint whether emotional eating is a problem for you is to keep a food journal for a couple of days. In addition to jotting down what you've eaten, make a note about how you were feeling at the time. Keeping such records can help you to determine how often you are eating for reasons other than hunger and to discover what types of foods you tend to turn to at these times. (Think chocolate!)

Researchers have discovered that dieting can cause you to lose your ability to recognize and respond to subtle appetite-related cues. If you're a veteran dieter, you may have gotten into the habit of allowing your body to become overly hungry and/or of ignoring your body's signs that it's had enough to eat. Here are some tips on teaching your body how to recognize these important cues—something that can help you to normalize your eating habits:

- Learn to recognize your own signals and be prepared to make a preemptive strike by feeding your body before it becomes totally ravenous. (If you wait too long before eating, you'll be so hungry that you'll be tempted to overeat.) As a rule of thumb, you can expect to experience one or more of the following types of symptoms when your body starts sending out an SOS for food: difficulty concentrating, feelings of faintness, headaches, irritability, light-headedness, and/or a mild gurgling or gnawing in the stomach.

Food for Thought

Don't be surprised if high-sugar, high-fat foods like chocolate top your list of foods that you turn to when the emotional eating monster rears it ugly head. Researchers believe that some emotional eating is triggered by a chemical imbalance in the brain: a deficiency in a brain chemical called serotonin that makes us feel calm and relaxed. Because carbohydrate-rich foods such as cakes, cookies, ice cream, and—of course—chocolate can temporarily boost your serotonin levels, some of us tend to reach for these foods because of their tranquilizing effects.

The Skinny

Work a variety of tastes and textures into each meal. This will boost your enjoyment of eating—something that can help to head off that urge to come back for seconds and thirds!

- Don't set yourself up for an episode of overeating. Rather than racing through your dinner, stop and appreciate each bite. This won't merely increase your enjoyment of your meal—something that will discourage you from coming back for a snack an hour after you're finished eating—it will also give your body a chance to alert you to the fact that it's full before you've shovelled in twice as much food as you need.

- Don't make it too easy for yourself to reach for seconds. Leave the serving dishes on the stove or the counter rather than putting them on the kitchen table. That will buy you a few extra minutes to decide whether you want more food because you're still hungry or whether you simply want to eat because the food is there.

- Eat balanced meals. Researchers have discovered that you are less likely to be satisfied with a meal that is heavy in some nutrients, but lacking in others—something that can cause you to head back into the kitchen because you're dissatisfied with the meal you just ate and not because you're hungry.

- Don't put anything in your mouth without asking yourself whether you're actually hungry or whether you want to eat because you're angry, depressed, bored, or simply too busy to take care of your needs in other ways. (If I'm tempted to reach for a high-fat food, I ask myself whether I'd still be hungry if I was reaching for broccoli instead!)

Are You Ready to Sign a Truce with Your Trigger Foods?

We all have trigger foods—foods that can very easily push us down the slippery slope called overeating. For me, it's oven-fresh white bread slathered in butter. Forget about eating a single slice—I could devour the entire loaf!

Sometimes it's possible to sign a truce with your trigger food—to come up with a game plan for controlling the amount of that food you eat. One woman I know is able to avoid the temptation to hit the Tim Horton's drive-thru on a daily basis because she knows that she's set aside enough calories in her

The Skinny

Are you tempted to pig out the night before you start a weight-loss program? That's because you're still thinking like a dieter. Rather than stuffing yourself with chocolate bars, potato chips, and other "forbidden" foods, remind yourself that these foods aren't going to fall off the face of the earth just because you're trying to lose weight. I mean, the last time I checked, there wasn't exactly a world-wide shortage of Twinkies!

food plan to indulge in a chocolate-dipped donut once a week.

That strategy doesn't work for everyone, however. Some women find that they're better off parting ways with their trigger foods entirely—banishing those foods from their lives until they feel like they'll be less likely to succumb to their charms. If you've had problems with a particular food for years, you might decide to go this route. (Perhaps your trigger food is simply the caloric equivalent to a Mr. Wrong—a food you can't say no to even though you know it's doing bad things to your head!)

Are You Ready to Stop "Thinking like a Dieter"?

One of the easiest ways to sabotage your weight-loss success is to insist on thinking like a dieter. Don't know what I mean? Let me explain. Dieters are notorious for their black-and-white thinking. They're either on a diet or they're off. The food that they're eating is either good or bad. There's never any in-between.

Unfortunately, you can only live with those types of perfectionistic standards for so long and when you fall off the wagon, it can be darned near impossible to get back on. The moral of the story? Lose the diet mentality!

That's a lesson that Margaret has learned the hard way: "I think I've become overwhelmed at times with having to do everything right, and not forgiving myself when I didn't. What helps me now is realizing that I have to change my eating habits forever, not just while I'm on a 'diet.' I will continue to have setbacks, but I need to stay focused on the goal of healthy eating for the rest of my life."

The Skinny

Buy yourself clothes that feel good right now rather than postponing any wardrobe purchases until the scale flashes some magic number. Why put off shopping until tomorrow when your wardrobe could be better today?

The Seven Secrets of Naturally Skinny Women

Have you ever wondered what makes naturally slim women different from the rest of us full-figured gals? So have I. In an effort to find out why these women seem to be able to eat cheesecake and anything else they want without ever gaining an ounce, I have spent years observing them in their natural habitats—the kitchen and the gym. Here's what I have discovered.

1 Naturally Skinny Women Know How to Put Food in Its Place

Naturally skinny women eat to live. They don't live to eat. In fact, sometimes they even forget to eat because they're so caught up with other things in their lives! They've learned how to put food in its place rather than giving it the white-glove treatment.

2 Naturally Skinny Women Know How to Have Fun at a Party

Naturally skinny women don't think that having fun has to be about eating. It's not that they spend more time swinging from the chandeliers or dancing around with lamp shades on their heads than the rest of us. It's just that they find other ways to spend their time than grazing at the buffet.

3 Naturally Skinny Women Don't Understand the Concept of Forbidden Foods

Naturally skinny women eat what they like and they don't eat what they don't like. This eliminates the need to pig out on "bad foods" or to force-feed themselves "good foods." They would also never dream of eating faux foods like low-fat muffins when they've got their hearts set on the real thing. They'd rather do without than settle for second best.

4 Naturally Skinny Women Know When It's Time to Put Down Their Forks

Naturally skinny women don't eat one more bite of food than they want. If they feel full in the middle of eating a piece of the most decadent and most expensive piece of cheesecake in the history of the world, they simply put down their forks. They don't see the point of eating when they are no longer hungry.

⑤ Naturally Skinny Women Know How to Enjoy Their Food

Naturally skinny women don't feel guilty about eating. They're not embarrassed to eat a huge piece of pie if they've got room for it, nor are they reluctant to order the "man-sized" serving of roast beef, even if the waiter looks startled when they place their order. In other words, they know how to enjoy their food.

The Skinny

"Studies have shown that the most satisfaction from eating comes from the first and last few bites and that the middle bites are automatic."

— Linda Omichinski, *You Count, Calories Don't*

⑥ Naturally Skinny Women Understand What Food Can and Can't Do for Them

Naturally skinny women don't view food as a "miracle cure" for whatever happens to be troubling them at the time. They know that cheesecake can't mend a broken heart and that a cheeseburger won't do a thing to make up for a missed promotion at work. They see food as the fuel that keeps their bodies running—nothing more and nothing less.

The Skinny

"That box of Oreos at your side may be your attempt to soothe and gratify yourself because you aren't taking care of your own needs. And it does—temporarily. But while eating is nurturing, especially when the foods are healthful, overeating is not: it destroys your body, and I don't have to tell you about the psychological ramifications."

— Janis Jibrin, *The Unofficial Guide to Dieting Safely*

⑦ Naturally Skinny Women Know How to Tell When They're Hungry and When They're Not

Naturally skinny women know how to read their bodies' signals. They know how to tell when their bodies need to be fed and when their bodies are already full. They listen to these signals and respond accordingly.

Now that we've talked about how you go about deciding whether you're ready to lose weight and considered what it's like to have a healthy relationship with food, let's move on and talk about another important ingredient in the recipe for weight loss: putting your support system in place.

6

Sister Act

"I'm sure it's possible to lose weight on your own," says Tammie, who is currently trying to lose weight, "but it is so much more pleasant to have a friend along for the ride. It makes the bad times easier to deal with if you have someone to call on for help. It holds you accountable to yourself: you have to answer to someone else when you goof up. It makes the good times even better: you have someone to laugh with, to cry with, and to jump for joy with!"

Imagine what it would be like to have someone cheering you on throughout your entire weight-loss journey: someone who would celebrate the milestone achievements with you and convince you to hang tough if temptation (a.k.a. The Chocolate Monster) reared its ugly head.

Believe it or not, that type of weight-loss support is pretty much yours for the asking. You simply need to know where to find it. That's what we're going to be talking about in the next part of this book.

Support Unlimited

Looking for weight-loss support? There's plenty of it out there. If you're someone who enjoys participating in groups, you might want to join a weight-loss support group. If you're not into the whole support-group scene, however, you might prefer to hook up with an individual weight-loss support person instead.

Group Weight-Loss Support

Group weight-loss support is great if you're a group kind of person—someone who has no trouble at all pouring out her soul to complete strangers or confessing her dietary sins to a room full of people, someone who will be motivated by (rather than intimidated by) the successes of other group members. On the other hand, it's not such a great option for you if you would find it difficult to fit a weekly meeting into your already insanely busy life or if you would feel awkward and embarrassed discussing your weight problems with people you barely know.

Before you sign up for any type of group weight-loss support, you'll want to find out as much as possible about the group in order to ensure that it's a good fit for you. Here are some questions you'll want to ask:

- **What is the group's philosophy?** Is this philosophy compatible with your own weight-loss goals? The last thing you want to do is to join a group where you feel pushed to lose more weight than you feel comfortable losing or that doesn't recommend the same approach to weight loss as you intend to use (e.g., a balance of healthy eating and physical activity).
- **What does it cost to join this group?** While some weight-loss support groups are free or almost-free, if you're signing up for a commercial weight-loss program, you will be expected to pay a weekly meeting fee whether or not you're actually able to attend that week's meeting. There can also be a variety of hidden costs—everything from packaged foods to weight-loss supplements to registration fees—so be sure to go into any such arrangements with your eyes wide open.
- **Are the meeting times convenient for you?** You're not going to get much benefit out of belonging to a weight-loss group if you're only able to attend meetings sporadically. When you're choosing a group, look for one that meets at times that will work for you—perhaps a workplace-based group that

The Skinny

The biggest drawback to turning to a commercial weight-loss program for weight-loss support is the cost. In addition to paying a weekly membership fee, you may also be required to purchase packaged foods, vitamin supplements, and other products. If you're considering this type of program, make sure you go in with your eyes wide open. Otherwise, you stand to lose something other than weight: cold, hard cash!

Food for Thought

"People who are truly supportive aren't those who scold you for that second piece of pie. Supportive people empathize with your weight loss struggle, usually because they've been there themselves."

— Janis Jibrin, *The Unofficial Guide to Dieting Safely*

will allow you to attend meetings during your lunch hour or an online group that you can participate in at any time of day or night.

- **What is the group's track record for success?** It's always a good idea to try to find out what percentage of people have lost weight as a result of participating in the group and what percentage have managed to maintain their weight loss over time (ideally, three to five years minimum). After all, there's no point in hooking up with a group that's batting zero!

- **Will the group also provide you with support after you reach your goal?** You'll also want to ask what happens when you reach your goal weight. Will you be able to continue to participate in the group or will you have to seek out another source of support at that point?

If you can't find a ready-made group that's to your liking, you might consider starting your own weight-loss support group. You could organize a group at work and arrange to meet once a week during your lunch hour, you could get a group of friends together at your house one night a week, or you could organize your own online weight-loss support group by starting a message board or mailing list and inviting other people to join. (See Appendix C for details on finding weight-loss support online.)

You can find a more detailed discussion of the pros and cons of various group weight-loss options in Table 6.1 on pages 90 and 91.

One-on-One Support

Wondering where you can find one-on-one weight-loss support? If you're really lucky, you might find it under your very own roof—either from your spouse or another family member. Otherwise, you may have to look a little farther afield. Either way, you'll want to find someone who's up to the job:

- **Someone who's committed to losing weight herself.** There's no doubt about it: the ideal weight-loss support person is someone who is either currently trying to lose weight or who has recently lost weight herself. While other people in your life who've never struggled with their weight can certainly provide you with plenty of encouragement, they won't be able to relate to what you're going through as much as someone who's a veteran of the Battle of the Bulge. There's just one small bit of fine print you need to be aware of if you decide to choose someone who is still in the weight-loss trenches: you need to make sure that she is every bit as committed to losing weight as you are. Nothing can short-circuit your weight-loss program more quickly, after all, than having your weight-loss buddy throw in the towel.

- **Someone who will motivate, not nag, you.** While you want someone who will force you to be accountable and who will encourage you to stay on track, the last thing you want to do is to recruit someone who will take that as a licence to play drill sergeant. It's friendly encouragement you're after—not the boot camp experience!

- **Someone who's both reliable and available.** You need a weight-loss support person who will be there for you through both thick and thin—someone who has the time to spend holding your hand and encouraging you to do battle with your nemesis, the Dairy Queen Peanut Buster Parfait. This probably rules out both your friend who's in medical school and your cousin who just had triplets. As much as they might like to be there for you, they simply don't have the time.

- **Someone who won't be threatened by your success.** It's important to choose a support person who will be happy about rather than threatened by your weight-loss success. (Hint: If you and your sister have been competing for grades in school, for boyfriends, and for Mom and Dad's attention since you were little kids, she's probably not your best choice for a weight-loss buddy!)

Wondering where to find such a weight-loss support person? Here are a few places to look:

- **Across the breakfast table.** Believe it or not, the weight-loss support person of your dreams might also be the man of your dreams. Studies have

Food for Thought

The dropout rate for exercise is three times higher when spouses are negative or indifferent toward their partner's commitment to exercise rather than when they are supportive.

The Skinny

"The last two times I tried to lose weight, it was for the men in my life, and it was never good enough for them. This time, I have a supportive boyfriend who loved me at 278 pounds, loves me at 233 pounds and will still love me no matter what size I am. This time, the only pressure to lose weight is coming from myself."

— Krista, who has lost over 50 pounds over the past year

TABLE 6.1

WHERE TO FIND THE SUPPORT YOU NEED

TYPE OF SUPPORT	PROS	CONS
Group Support		
Commercial weight-loss programs	*Support and motivation.* You will have the opportunity to meet face-to-face with other people who are struggling to lose weight or to meet with a weight-loss counsellor who will encourage you to stick with your program.	*Cost.* In addition to paying a weekly membership fee, you may also be required to purchase packaged foods, vitamin supplements, and other products. *Scheduling.* You have to be able to fit a weekly meeting or counselling session into your schedule. *Philosophy/program.* You may or may not agree with the group's philosophy or be prepared to stick with the prescribed weight-loss program. *No opportunity for anonymity.* If you feel awkward discussing your weight problems with others, you may want to consider opting for some other form of weight-loss support instead.
Non-profit groups (e.g., Take Off Pounds Sensibly or Overeaters Anonymous)	*Support and motivation.* You will have the opportunity to meet face-to-face with other people who are struggling to lose weight or to change their relationship with food. *Relatively inexpensive.* Unlike commercial weight-loss programs, non-profit groups tend to run on a cost-recovery basis, something that can make them extremely affordable.	*Scheduling.* You have to be able to fit a weekly meeting into your schedule. *Philosophy/program.* You may or may not agree with the group's philosophy. Overeaters Anonymous, for example, is a 12-step program that treats overeating as an addiction—a viewpoint you may or may not share. *No opportunity for anonymity.* If you feel awkward discussing your weight problems with others, you may want to consider opting for some other form of weight-loss support instead.

shown that women whose partners support their weight-loss efforts are far more likely to be successful than women whose partners are indifferent to or who go to great lengths to sabotage their weight-loss efforts. Unfortunately, these supportive guys are a relatively rare breed: a Harvard Medical School study showed that only one-third of women are able to obtain this type of support from their partners.

- **Within your family or your circle of friends.** One of the best ways to find a weight-loss support person is to offer to be someone else's weight-loss support person. If you know someone else who is trying to lose weight (perhaps a family member or a friend), why not suggest that the two of you

| Online support groups (message boards, e-mail lists, chat rooms, etc.) | *Scheduling.* You can participate in the weight-loss group as much or as little as your schedule permits, and you don't have to participate at any fixed time of day or night. You can simply read your e-mail or post to the message board whenever you have some free time. (Note: If your online weight group meets via chat room, you will have to ensure that you're able to participate in the online chats at the appropriate time.)

Cost. There are plenty of excellent online support groups that you can join free of charge.

Anonymity. If you are embarrassed by your weight problems, you can post your comments anonymously or under a pseudonym. You also don't have to worry about anyone saying anything nasty about your appearance—a significant concern for women who have large amounts of weight to lose.

No geographical limitations. You can tap into this type of support no matter where you live, provided that you have access to the Internet. | *Dealing with strangers.* Some people find it difficult to seek support from complete strangers, particularly since the anonymity of the Internet allows people to conceal as much information as they want about themselves.

An uncertain track record for success. Most of these groups are fairly informal, so it's unlikely that you'll be able to find out much about the group's track record for success. |

One-on-One Support

| One-on-one support from a weight-loss buddy | *Cost.* This type of support is generally free. (The only exception, of course, is if you sign up for a commercial weight-loss program that includes one-on-one counselling sessions or you hire a dietitian or psychologist to provide you with one-on-one support.)

Scheduling. The two of you can come up with a support arrangement that will fit into both of your schedules (e.g., exercising together or providing daily support via e-mail). | *Privacy.* There isn't the same opportunity for anonymity as there is with an online support group, but there's more privacy than what you would normally find in a weight-loss support group. |

offer support to one another? You don't necessarily have to be in the same part of the country, by the way: a daily e-mail can be just as motivating as a daily telephone call.

- **At work.** Know someone else at work who's having trouble resisting the call of the vending machine? Why not join forces and offer some on-the-job weight-loss support to one another?

The Skinny

- **Online.** If you spend much time at online weight-loss message boards, you're bound to strike up a friendship with some of the folks you meet there. Why not see if any of them are interested in e-mailing back and forth to offer daily support? I'm in regular e-mail contact with a lot of women I've met this way and it really helps to keep me on track.

The Benefits of Reaching Out for Support

There's no doubt about it: reaching out for support can make it a lot easier to stick with a weight-loss program. Here are just a few of the benefits you can expect to experience as a result of reaching out for support:

- **Reassurance that you're not the only one fighting this battle.** If most of your friends are within 10 pounds of their ideal weight, you may feel like you're the only one with a weight problem. It can be reassuring to discover that there are plenty of other women in the same boat as you. Krista notes, "I feel a real connection with these people as they are facing the same problems as I am. I don't think I could have come quite so far without knowing just how many others there are out there struggling through the same things I face every day."
- **The opportunity to focus—and re-focus—on your weight-loss goals.** Ann (another Incredible Shrinking Ann!) starts and ends each day by visiting a particular online weight-loss message board because doing so helps to keep her focused on her goals.
- **Motivation to stick with your program when you're tempted to do anything but.** Elizabeth credits her e-mail buddies with helping her to stay on track on her good, bad, and ugly days: "You get personal encouragement if you need it, pats on the back when you do well, and a helping hand when you stumble." Shari also gives her online weight-loss group full credit for helping her to deal with her emotional eating problems: "Our expectations for ourselves and one another are high and my recovery from compulsive eating is directly tied to my relationship with the group."

- **Someone to share your successes with.** Perhaps the best reason of all to line up some weight-loss support is so that you'll have someone to share your successes with along the way. Krista says, "There is nothing more satisfying than knowing you have so many cheerleaders out there who truly care about your success and your commitment."

The Skinny

"In one of the groups I belonged to, the people talked so much about cheating that it was almost like the thing to do. The group ended up being a bad influence on me. I tried four groups before I found the two I am with now, so keep trying if you don't find a good one at first."

— Catherine, who is currently losing weight

7

The First Week Survival Guide

Planning to write your law school admissions test, to head to the altar, or to have a baby in the near future? No problem. You can sign up for special classes that will prepare you for each of these momentous events.

Thinking of losing weight? Sorry, girlfriend. The one thing you won't find advertised on the grocery store bulletin board is weight-loss preparation classes. (It's a darned shame, too! Imagine how helpful it would be if you could sign up for classes that would teach you how to use relaxation breathing techniques to get through even the most intense chocolate craving and that would also educate your partner about the importance of catering to the every whim of a woman in your "condition"!)

In this chapter, we're going to boldly go where no other weight-loss book has gone before. We're going to talk about what you can expect during the first week of a new weight-loss program: the good, the bad, and the ugly. We'll start out by talking about the key challenges that you will face when you're getting started and what you can do to overcome them. Then we'll zero in on what I like to call the "17 Habits of Highly Successful Losers"—first-week survival tips from women who have lost weight and lived to tell!

The Truth About the First Week

Think every woman who's losing weight looks as euphoric as the woman in the Jenny Craig commercial—you know, the woman who's so excited about weighing in that she practically breaks into a sprint?

Time for a reality check. While losing weight doesn't have to be an exercise in torture (unless, of course, you go for a very low-calorie diet plan), no weight-loss program is entirely free of challenges. What ads of the Jenny Craig variety invariably fail to tell you is that there are rough spots in every weight-loss program—times when it's all you can do not to abandon your weight-loss program to run off with Colonel Sanders or the Dickie Dee Ice Cream Man!

The first week tends to be particularly challenging for most of us. In fact, it can make or break you. Here's why:

- You don't stand to lose much by throwing in the towel. Now matter how committed you are to your new weight-loss program, it takes time for the pounds to come off and the inches to disappear. Until that starts to happen, it's easy to become discouraged and pack it in in the towel. After all, at this point, you haven't got much to lose. The way around this particular problem is to sign up for a crash course in patience! The extra pounds didn't show up overnight, so they aren't going to disappear overnight either. Bottom line? If you're serious about losing weight, you have to be prepared to invest time and effort before you start seeing the payoff.

- It's tempting to slip back into old habits. Are you in the habit of snacking in front of the TV set? Don't be surprised if you catch yourself going into automatic eating mode from time to time: grabbing a handful of chips and a can of pop before you even realize what you're doing. This morning—eight months into my weight-loss program!—I automatically reached for a glass and was about to pour myself a huge glass of orange juice when I remembered that I don't drink fruit juice anymore. (I prefer to sit down and enjoy a piece of fruit rather than knocking back a glass of juice in a matter of seconds.) As you can see, it's not the least bit unusual to forget your new eating habits and switch into auto-pilot mode from time to time.

The Skinny

Are you in the habit of eating while you're cooking? Here's an easy way to break the habit. Pop a piece of chewing gum into your mouth so that you will have to think twice before you start nibbling. (You're unlikely to want to pop a piece of cheese or pasta into your mouth when you're chewing a piece of cinnamon-flavoured gum!) You could save yourself hundreds of calories by reaching for that stick of gum—calories that you won't particularly enjoy anyway. After all, how much dining pleasure can you get out of a snack that's consumed while you're leaning over the stove or the kitchen sink?

The Skinny

"I let myself enjoy whatever it is I want. However, I do nothing else but eat that item. I limit my portion and slowly, intently focus on every bit, on every flavour and texture, and on totally enjoying the whole experience. That usually satisfies my craving. I've found that I can usually feel satisfied by eating one half of a donut rather than the whole dozen."

— Dawnette, who is now within 10 pounds of her goal weight

- You may find yourself craving some of your favourite foods. If your favourite foods are high-sugar or high-fat goodies like donuts, potato chips, and ice cream (and, frankly, whose aren't?), you could find yourself experiencing some powerful cravings until your body becomes accustomed to a new way of eating. While your taste in food will change over time—believe it or not, the day will come when you will no longer particularly like the greasy taste and texture of fried chicken or nachos—it takes time to retrain your taste buds. In the meantime, you need to be prepared to do battle with your cravings. Some women deal with their cravings by having a small serving of the foods they crave; others find that doing so only prolongs the agony of withdrawal, so they prefer to go "cold turkey." You'll have to experiment a little to find out which solution works best for you. (We'll be returning to this point again later in this chapter.)

- You may feel so irritable that you may start to wonder if losing weight is actually worth the effort. Even if you don't chop your food consumption drastically—a guaranteed way of putting yourself in one ugly mood—you can still expect to feel a bit irritable during the early weeks of your weight-loss program. Irritability is more likely to be a problem for women who are emotional eaters. After all, if you're used to using food as a sedative—turning to food for comfort whenever you're having a bad day—you can expect to experience some major symptoms of "withdrawal" when you force your body to find other ways of coping with the highs and lows of day-to-

The Skinny

"If I have a craving, I try to distract myself. I empty the dishwasher or straighten up something in the house to get my mind off food. Substituting doesn't work well for me. For example, if I really want chocolate, eating carrots isn't going to help.

"My advice is to eat what you crave, but just eat a tiny bit of it. Have a bit of chocolate. Go out and buy a piece of good chocolate and eat it out of the house. Don't bring a bunch of chocolate home, where you might run into trouble. Give yourself what you want, but control how much of it you eat. I found that ignoring the craving can lead to an obsession and a binge for me."

— Margaret, who is currently trying to lose weight

day life. Fortunately, these effects tend to be short-lived, provided you learn new ways of managing the stress of daily living. As you start developing other coping skills—going for a walk around the block or picking up the phone to call a friend, you'll stop being so dependent on food and you'll start feeling a little saner.

- You may find your energy level lagging a little. If you're used to using food as a source of instant energy (e.g., you reach for a Mars bar or donut each afternoon in order to give yourself a temporary energy burst), you may feel a bit dragged out when you first kick your sugar habit. Fortunately, your energy level will start to pick up once your body gets hooked on healthier foods and you start exercising regularly. (Yes, Virginia, there is an exercise boost associated with being physically active!) You can help yourself to get over this temporary energy slump by marrying protein to carbohydrates at each meal and by turning to high-fibre carbohydrates whenever possible. Rather than having a bare naked multigrain bagel for breakfast or lunch, dress it up with some low-fat cheese, a bit of egg salad, or a slice of turkey. The payoff to working some protein into each meal can be considerable: instead of experiencing a mid-morning or mid-afternoon slump, you'll be able to hang in there for a good two to three hours before your energy level begins to crash and your stomach starts alerting your brain that it's time to eat again. This simple trick can literally change your life. It has certainly changed mine. (Yes, girlfriend, I'm a Born Again Protein Eater!)

- You may experience a few aches and pains when you first start to become physically active. If you haven't been exercising for a very long time, you'll likely get some aches and pains when you first start hitting the gym. It's not surprising that this happens, of course: you're asking certain muscle groups to get back to work after a prolonged vacation! In most cases, these aches and

Food for Thought

Do you think of yourself as a chocolate junkie or a cheesecake addict? You might not be too far off the mark. According to Dr. Stephen Gullo, author of *Thin Tastes Better: Control Your Food Triggers Without Feeling Deprived*, it is possible to be "hooked" on certain types of foods. "Food cravings aren't all in your mind. You crave foods because your body 'remembers' the physiological effect the food had on you when you consumed it in the past. In fact, research has shown that the foods we perceive as enjoyable or rewarding actually activate the same 'reward pathways' in the brain that are triggered by certain drugs of abuse—like cocaine. When you experience a 'food flash,' you are really experiencing a milder form of the drug cravings that affect recovering addicts."

Fat Chance

Tempted to cut back on the amount of protein in your diet because it's "too fattening"? Think again. Not only does protein weigh in at a relatively skinny four calories per gram, a Laval University study showed that people who get enough protein in their diet eat 164 fewer calories per day than those who don't, because protein leaves them feeling satisfied longer. The secret to making protein work for, not against, you is to seek out low-fat sources of protein and not to go overboard when it comes to portion sizes. Despite what some of the high-protein diet gurus would like you to believe, you can have too much of a good thing.

pains don't amount to much more than a little stiffness or muscle soreness the next day. What's more, they tend to be relatively short-lived, disappearing as your fitness level improves. Until then, you can minimize them by stretching both before and after your workout (see Chapter 4, "Gym Class Revisited") and by easing into your fitness routine gradually. In other words, it's not a good idea to go from being totally inactive to signing up for an advanced aerobics class at your local gym!

The 17 Habits of Highly Successful Losers

Wondering what separates the winners from the losers—what allows some women to achieve their weight-loss goals while others decide to call it quits? You're about to find out! While researching this book, I had the opportunity to interview a number of women who have successfully won the Battle of the Bulge. Here's their best advice on getting your weight-loss program off to the strongest possible start.

(1) Know Thyself

I've said it before and I'll say it again: there's no such thing as a one-size-fits-all weight-loss program. You increase your odds of sticking to your program if you custom fit it to your own life. That means understanding what will and won't work for you on both the eating and exercise fronts.

Amy, who recently lost 67 pounds, decided early on in her weight-loss program that she wasn't cut out for any sort of starvation diet. Therefore boosting her activity level would be critical to her success. "I absolutely love food, so nothing that restricts food too severely works for me," she explains. "I've found that what works best for me is exercise (lots!) and food in moderation."

Heather took a radically different approach to exercise when she designed her weight-loss program. She concluded that she'd be tempted to abandon her program altogether if she tried to make too many changes too soon. "I wanted to spend my time and energy regaining control over myself where food was concerned," she explains. "I 'let' myself not exercise so that I would only have to focus on one area at a time. I think that is one of the main reasons people can't diet successfully: they think that they have to wake up tomorrow, jog five miles, eat perfectly, drink lots of water, and not have a single cookie. It's too much at once and it's too overwhelming. It's the classic all-or-nothing mentality. They don't realized that they can spend a few weeks learning to drink water every day—and that when they're comfortable with that, they can start walking 20 minutes a day—and then, after a few weeks, they can start making food changes. It doesn't have to be all at the same time."

> ## The Skinny
>
> "I think you need to research and devise your own weight-loss program if you're going to lose weight successfully and keep it off. It's not about following some plan that may not be right for everybody. You have to find what's right for you."
>
> — Kathryn, who recently lost 70 pounds

② Plan to Be Successful

There's a reason why the banks are more likely to fork over the cash for your new business venture if you've written a business plan: they know that entrepreneurs who plan for their success are far more likely to achieve their business goals than those who choose to fly by the seat of their pants. The same thing applies to weight loss: you're far more likely to be successful at losing weight if you plan ahead than if you decide to wing the whole weight loss thing.

Now before you accuse me of taking kick-backs from all my friends in the corporate writing business, hear me out! No one's suggesting that you set aside a few weeks of your life to draft a formal, 75-page weight-loss plan (although, frankly, my sister the M.B.A. might not think that's such a bad idea!). What you do need to do, however, is to put together a game plan that will help you to deal with—or, ideally, avoid—the types of weight-loss problems that might otherwise short-circuit your success. Here are a few examples:

- **Running out of healthy foods.** In a perfect world, we would all find time to grocery shop on a regular basis, thereby ensuring that we'd never run out of fresh produce and other weight-loss program essentials. Unfortunately, the world is anything but perfect (unless, of course, your name happens to be Martha Stewart): a deadline at work, a sick kid, or a car that's on the fritz can prevent you from making your regular pilgrimage to the grocery store. That's why it's important to keep a variety of weight-loss-friendly canned goods on hand at all times. That way, if you can't make it to the grocery store to pick up

The Skinny

"If I have the right food around, I can make the right choices. If I don't, I'll eat what's there. It's a no-brainer, but I have to make the time to do it. Unfortunately, I don't always do it in time!"

— Margaret, who is currently trying to lose weight

fresh fruit, salad ingredients, and lean ground beef, you can fall back on your in-house stash of unsweetened applesauce, canned tomatoes, and water-packed tuna instead. (If you don't have these kinds of healthy foods on hand, you'll find yourself faced with the mind-warping challenge of making a healthy dinner out of cream of mushroom soup, Kraft Dinner, and instant pudding. Best of luck!)

- **Playing Russian roulette in the grocery store.** Want to play a fun game of chance with your weight-loss program? Here's how to play. Rather than planning ahead and shopping from a grocery list, wander up and down the grocery store aisles filling your cart with anything that happens to catch your eye, whether the food in question is good, bad, or downright ugly. Do those cupcakes look yummy? Pop 'em in your cart. Can't resist those cheese-flavoured Doritos? Don't even try! There's room in your cart for at least a couple of bags. Tempted to inhale all the ooey-gooey cheese spreads in the deli department? Start inhaling away. Finding that your willpower is getting in the way and stopping you from succumbing to temptation? Shop on an empty stomach! That should make the game a little more challenging. As you can see, you drastically increase your odds of sabotaging your weight-loss program if you leave your grocery shopping to chance. Why play Russian roulette with your weight program when there's a smarter alternative: planning ahead!

- **Forgetting to pack a lunch if you're going to have an insanely busy day.** We all have crazy days: days when the only thing that even remotely resembles a "break" is the 15 minutes you spend in the car driving your kid to a hockey practice. On days like these, it can be hard to find time to stop for a meal—that's why it's important to plan ahead. If you've got a piece of fruit and a turkey sandwich in your purse, you'll be less likely to pull into the nearest Tim Horton's drive-thru when the hunger pangs inevitably strike. This is definitely one of those cases when an ounce of prevention is worth a pound of cure!

- **Leading yourself into temptation.** Unless you're some sick kind of masochist who likes inflicting pain on herself, you wouldn't think of forcing yourself to sit in front of a plate of freshly baked chocolate chip cookies. (The temptation would simply be too great for all but the superheroes among us!) Believe it or not, you may be leading yourself into similar temptation simply by failing to plan ahead. How often have you arrived at a dinner party only to realize that the hostess isn't serving a single healthy entrée? Or discovered to your horror that every single roadside restaurant along the 401 specializes in dishing up the types of high-fat foods that you'd really prefer to avoid? The way to avoid setting yourself up for temptation and failure is to master the art of planning ahead: show up at the dinner party with a low-fat entrée in hand or pack a healthy lunch that you can enjoy in the parking lot of one of those roadside chambers of horror.

> ### The Skinny
>
> Is the food court at the mall your downfall? Change your shopping route so that you can bypass the food area entirely or decide in advance what low-fat snack you're going to treat yourself to if you're dying for a snack. Hint: You can usually find a garden salad, fresh fruit, and low-fat milk if you hunt hard enough!

- **Packing a deadly weapon.** You might not think of a pocketful of change as a deadly weapon, but it can be if you put it to ill use. If you know that you're vulnerable to the vending machines at work, take a lesson from successful loser Kathryn and leave your extra change at home.
- **Failing to cheat-proof your surroundings.** One of the simplest and most effective ways to plan for your success is to cheat-proof your surroundings. You're less likely to indulge in your after-dinner munchies habit if you have to hop in your car and head for the closest variety store in order to get your "fix" of chips. If you absolutely have to keep some treats on hand because other people in your family might stage a mutiny if you were to declare your home a treat-free zone, then at least be smart about it. Buy foods that they love, but that you can live without. That's why you'll find my fridge stocked with (yuck!) root beer and my cupboards stocked with (gag!) ketchup-flavoured potato chips: my kids love these foods, but I wouldn't be caught dead eating this stuff.
- **Not having enough emergency dinners on hand.** We all have days when we arrive home from work too tired to do anything but hit the automatic dial button for Pizza Pizza. The way to avoid falling into this particular trap is to ensure that you've got a smorgasbord of equally appealing prepared dinners sitting in your freezer. You can either rely on commercially prepared products (my favourite is President's Choice Mexican Bean Casserole) or you can turn your own kitchen into a frozen food factory. (All you need is a pantry

The Skinny

full of low-fat cookbooks and casserole dishes. You'll find some of my favourite cookbooks listed in Appendix E.) If you're not much of a cook, but don't particularly like the "packaged" taste of frozen dinners, you might want to do what veteran "loser" Jill does when she finds herself hit with a dinnertime emergency: she adds some pizzazz to commercial frozen dinners by throwing in some spices and stir-fried veggies. "It takes all of ten minutes to do," she confides.

(3) Focus on Your Weight-Loss Goals

Not sure why it's important to focus on your weight-loss goals? Any three-year-old would be happy to bring you up to speed by telling you the story of *The Little Engine That Could.* While you might feel a little silly walking around chanting "I think I can, I think I can," as that smart little locomotive did, you can certainly do the next best thing: find ways to revisit your weight-loss goals a couple of times each day.

Here are a few ideas:

- Start your day by reminding yourself why you're hoping to lose weight. If your life becomes a marathon event the moment your feet hit the bedroom floor, set your alarm clock to go off five minutes earlier so that you can reflect on your goals when you're still in bed. Or use the time in the shower when you're waiting for the creme rinse to work its magic to psych yourself up for a day of healthy eating and plenty of physical activity.

- Remind yourself of your weight-loss goals each time you open the refrigerator door. One successful loser I know claims that a visual picture of herself at her goal weight flashes through her head each time reaches for something to eat.

- If you're a visually minded person, you might want to try using photos to motivate yourself to achieve your weight-loss goals. I've got two photos of myself in plain sight of my desk: a photo of me at a svelte-for-me 142 pounds—and a photo of me at my all-time high of 256 pounds. Talk about motivation!

- Focus on your weight-loss goals in the evening before you go to bed. Psychologists have discovered that the problem-solving parts of our brains continue to work while we're sleeping—something that helps to explain why you can wake up in the morning and suddenly remember where your car keys are, even though you couldn't find them anywhere before you went to bed. Why not use this capability to your advantage when you're trying to lose weight? Who knows? Maybe you'll wake up in the morning with a brand new strategy for taming the chocolate monster.

④ Pamper Yourself

You've already mastered the art of pampering yourself with food. Now it's time to teach yourself some new tricks. Rather than reaching for some high-sugar, high-fat treat, challenge yourself to find food-free ways to pamper yourself. Over time, you'll stop viewing food as a reward and start seeing it for what it is: a fuel source for your body!

Can't remember the last time you pampered yourself with something other than food? Neither could I when I first started my weight-loss program. Fortunately, I've become a little more creative along the way. You can, too. Here's a list of some of my favourite food-free ways of pampering myself:

- Going to bed early. Sleep, glorious sleep. Can any woman ever have enough? I think not. One of my favourite ways to pamper myself is to hit the sack early—alone!
- Treating myself to a new book. I admit it. I'm a book addict. I can't get enough of them. I mean, not only do I like to write them: I enjoy reading them, too. One of my favourite ways to reward myself for the progress I've made toward my weight-loss goals is to tune out the chaos around me (no small feat, since I've got four kids) by diving into a new book.

The Skinny

Ignorance isn't bliss at all—at least not when it comes to weight loss. One sure way to boost your odds of achieving your weight-loss goals is to learn as much as possible about nutrition and exercise. Take a low-fat cooking class or read up on the hottest new trends in exercise. Not only are you likely to walk away with some new ideas that will help you to add sizzle to your menus and work-outs: you'll also have the chance to focus on your weight-loss goals at the same time.

The Skinny

Start treating yourself like a queen. Since knights in shining armour are in chronically short supply these days, you could be old and gray before anyone else gets around to treating you like royalty. So rather than waiting for some fairy-tale ending, just do it yourself. Set aside some time every day to do something you enjoy, whether that's soaking in a bubble bath, lounging on the couch reading a steamy novel, or gabbing on the phone with a friend.

The Skinny

Don't wait until you reach your goal weight to start looking your best. Here are some tips on dressing skinny:

- Streamline your body by dressing in a single colour. The darker the colour, the more dramatic the effect. (Guess this helps to explain the perennial appeal of the "little black dress.")

- Make your legs look longer and thinner by choosing pantyhose that's the same colour as your shoes. (Your legs will seem to go on forever.)

- Conceal tummy bulges by wearing loose-fitting vests or long jackets or by choosing pleated pants. (Just make sure that the pleats aren't overly full or you'll end up adding to— not subtracting from—your tummy.)

- Camouflage a chubby neck by opting for shirts and blouses with V-neck rather than rounded neck styles.

- Avoid clothing that's either too tight or too loose. Clothing that's too tight will reveal every bump and bulge (something that very few figures—slim or otherwise—can stand up to), while clothing that's too loose will make you look and feel bigger.

- Reading the newspaper. My print addiction extends beyond books, I must confess. There are few things I enjoy more than reading the morning newspaper—particularly on the weekend, when there are all those great extra sections to enjoy. It's hard to imagine anything else than can give you so much enjoyment for a buck.

- Having coffee with a friend. I hate to even think about how much money I've spent at Haaselton's— the gourmet coffee shop that I tend to frequent— but I suspect I probably underwrote the cost of the jazzy new frozen cappuccino machine they recently unveiled! I still can't believe that my beverage of choice—a decaffeinated latte made with low-fat milk—is 100% sin-free. Who says there isn't a Patron Saint of Dieters?

- Hitting the gym. A year ago, I would have burst out laughing if anyone had tried to convince me that working out at the gym could be considered a way of pampering yourself. Now it's the first thing I think of when I unexpectedly find myself with a block of time to myself (provided there's someone to watch my kids).

- Treating myself to a new item of clothing. For years and years, I avoided buying myself anything other than bargain-basement clothing because I was convinced that I was about to lose weight. Last year, I finally broke down and bought myself some drop-dead gorgeous clothes—clothes that made me feel like a million bucks even though I was still more than 100 pounds overweight. While I can't wear some of those clothes today because I've lost too much weight, I don't regret purchasing them at all. Those clothes made me feel attractive when I was at my heaviest, and while I was losing my first 50 pounds I figure it cost me about $200 to feel good for the six months when the outfits actually fit me—six months when I would otherwise have been stuck schlepping around in tent-style dresses and stretch pants. I don't know about you, but I think that $200 was a bargain.

- Treating myself at the beauty parlour. While I'm not one to go for manicures—typing eight hours a day is, after all, hell on one's nails—I do enjoy getting my hair coloured and styled on a regular basis. I usually leave the salon feeling like a princess. (I figure it's only a matter of time until I have a car accident on my way home. Let's just say I tend to spend a bit too much time admiring myself in the rear-view mirror after Tom has worked his usual magic.)

- Hitting the tub. There's nothing like an hour-long soak in the tub to make you feel like Queen for a Day. (Either that or a shrivelled prune.) My friend Jan (who hasn't got any weight to lose, but who is lovable nonetheless) has turned soaking in the jacuzzi into an art. She dims the lights, lights some candles, pours herself a glass of wine, and fills the tub with cascades of bubble bath. (Hey, if a mother of four like Jan can find time to do this, so can the rest of us!)

> ### The Skinny
>
> "I keep a list on the back of my clipboard of 25 of my favourite pastimes, such as visiting an antique mall, going to an antique bookstore, buying fresh flowers and painting them, sorting through my jewellery box, taking a long walk, inviting a friend to tea, writing a long letter to a friend, reading an old English novel, watching my favourite movie—in other words, something that feels like a delicious emotional treat to myself."
>
> — Ann, who is currently trying to lose weight

Note: You don't necessarily have to spend a lot of money in order to pamper yourself. Sometimes it's the little things—a cup of tea with a friend or a walk in the woods with your kids—that do the most for your mental health. Resist the temptation to simply switch addictions: to stop overeating and start overspending!

⑤ Avoid Boredom

One of the surest ways to doom your weight-loss program to failure is to bore yourself into quitting. That's why successful losers know that varying their eating and exercise routines is the key to staying on track.

Here are a few tips on spicing up your weight-loss program:

- Think outside the box when it comes to planning your menus. Don't assume that you can only have breakfast in the morning. Have it for dinner, too! Or start your day off with a zesty dish of low-fat pizza, if that's what appeals to you.

- Don't get in a rut when you're shopping for food. Next time you hit the grocery store, check out all the products on the shelf—not just the ones that you're used to picking up week after week.
- Try a new piece of exercise equipment the next time you hit the gym. It's an easy way to add more spice to your workout. Just one quick word of caution: make sure you ask someone to show you the ropes. Not only are you likely to burn fewer calories if you're using the equipment incorrectly—according to the experts, you burn approximately 7% fewer calories for each 10 pounds of body weight that you support by leaning on the equipment—you also run the risk of injuring yourself.
- Sign up for an exercise challenge at the gym or organize your own exercise challenge with a group of friends. (Hey, there's nothing like a bit of friendly competition to make you want to stick with your program!)

(6) Don't Let Food Control Your Life

Don't let your focus on healthy eating turn into an obsession with eating, period. It's easy to get so caught up with measuring and weighing your food and planning your menus that you don't think of anything other than food. Margaret found that the solution for her was to put her food scale away: "I felt too regimented and locked in," she recalls. "I wanted to rebel. I decided I'd rather estimate and find a way to moderate my portions without always weighing, measuring, and obsessing."

While it's important to plan ahead, it's also important to keep food in perspective. It's not the most important thing in your life. (Or, at least, it shouldn't be!) It's simply the fuel that allows your body to do a million-and-one wonderful things.

(7) Keep Yourself Honest

Are you prepared to tell the truth, the whole truth, and nothing but the truth? You should be. After all, the only one you're cheating by "forgetting" about the donut that you "accidentally" ate is yourself! If you find it tempting to be less than honest in admitting to yourself how many calories you're consuming over the course of a day, you might want to try putting yourself on the weight-loss world's equivalent to probation: keeping a weight-loss diary.

I'm not a great fan of food diaries—I think they tend to make you obsess about every bite of food that goes into your mouth—but they can help to keep you honest. (After all, you're likely to think twice before you knock back a thousand calories in M & Ms if you know you're going to have to come clean about it later on.) They can also help you to do a postmortem on any binges that happen to occur: you can look back on what you ate in the day or two leading up to the binge and see if it might have been triggered by something you ate—or didn't eat.

(8) Enjoy Each Bite of Food That You Put in Your Mouth

There's no law that says that you have to deprive your-self of the joy of eating just because you're trying to lose weight. (Or if there is such a law, neither of my two lawyer sisters has bothered to tell me about it.) I would argue, in fact, that you have a greater-than-usual need to enjoy your food when you're trying to lose weight, if only because you're consuming fewer calories.

Here are some tips on maximizing your EPM (Enjoyment Per Mouthful):

- Don't eat when you're distracted. Are you a master when it comes to uncon-scious eating—shovelling the food in while barely noticing what you're doing? You might fall into this all-too-common trap if you're in the habit of eating while you're reading, watching TV, or driving in the car. You suddenly real-ize to your horror that you've inhaled an entire box of Timbits and you can't even remember what flavours were in the box!
- Don't eat when there's chaos erupting all around you. How much do you enjoy your meals when you're arguing with your husband or trying to nego-tiate a cease-fire between two of your kids? Not a whole lot, if you're like me. I've found over the years that I get zero satisfaction out of calories that are eaten when I feel like strangling a family member. I'm far better off just

---

The Skinny

"I've learned that certain times of day are harder than others when it comes to having willpower. Right after dinner is my toughest time because I usually work out before dinner and am ravenous at dinnertime. Sometimes I'll keep eating even when I know I've had enough. The way I can combat this is by taking breaks mid-meal to make sure I know when I'm full. I stop eating and put my plate aside for ten minutes or so and then resume eating if I still feel hungry. I also try to drink plenty of water at this time, to fill me up."

— Kathryn, who has lost 70 pounds over the past year

putting down my fork and waiting for a momentary lull in the storm. Then I have at least a fighting chance of enjoying the food in front of me.

- Don't eat when you're standing up. Your enjoyment of a meal decreases considerably if you have to eat it when you're standing up. This is one of the reasons why it's easy to go back for plateful after plateful of cocktail food—far more than you'd ever consume if you were actually sitting down at a table.

- Get in the habit of making mealtimes special. Rather than saving your good china for your mother-in-law's annual visit, put it on the table today. Add some candles and fresh flowers and you'll feel like you're dining in the finest restaurant—at least until it's time to wash the dishes. (Note to mothers of toddlers: Don't skip this tip just because your two-year-old likes to treat dinner plates like frisbees. Studies have shown that children tend to be on their best behaviour at the dinner table when mealtimes are treated like special occasions. Besides, what have you got to lose other than a Royal Doulton plate or two?)

- Don't eat foods that you hate—even if they're good for you. There are enough foods on this planet that you should be able to eat nutritionally balanced meals without ever having to shovel down food that you totally detest. You could show up on my doorstep for dinner 365 days in a row and you would never—I repeat never—find Brussels sprouts, asparagus, liver, or kidney on the dinner menu.

- Don't pass on the foods you love just because they're a bit pricey. Before I get myself in trouble with all the financial planners out there, allow me to explain. I'm not suggesting that you should buy caviar on a tuna fish budget. I'm simply saying that you should be willing to splurge a little when it comes to adding healthy foods you enjoy to your diet. Let me give you an example. It was an accepted fact in my house when I was growing up that it was a sin to buy cantaloupes when they cost more than $0.99 per pound. (It was also considered to be a crime against humanity to buy bananas that cost more than $0.29 per pound or green grapes that cost more than $0.99 per pound. Yes, Mom and Dad certainly did their bit to teach us the value of a dollar!) As time went on, it became harder and harder to pick up fruit at

The Skinny

Think Martha Stewart is the only one capable of working magic in the kitchen? Why not try this little bit of culinary sleight-of-hand? Rather than smacking your entrée down on a standard-sized dinner plate, put it on a smaller-than-average-sized dinner plate instead. Your serving will look a lot more substantial. (Guess this is proof that size really does matter after all—at least when it comes to dinner plates.)

these prices. (Inflation was, after all, one of the ugly legacies of the 1970s—even uglier than hot pants and platform shoes!) To this day, a red light still goes off in my head when I pick up a cantaloupe that costs more than $0.99 a pound—but then I remind myself that it's actually a bargain when compared to high-priced packaged foods, many of which were responsible for my gaining weight in the first place. And when I factor in all the money I've spent on weight-loss products over the years, that cantaloupe becomes an absolute steal.

> ### The Skinny
>
> "In the beginning, the hunger is a good feeling for me. It makes me feel virtuous, even! But if I let myself get too hungry, that's when I get out of control and eat what's convenient rather than what's right. When I do get hungry, I eat mini carrots, yogurt, and fruit."
>
> — Margaret, who is trying to lose weight

⑨ Guard Against Hunger

Hunger is public enemy number one—at least in the weight-loss world. One of the easiest ways to fall off the healthy-eating wagon is to allow yourself to get so hungry that you become positively obsessed with food. (You can assume that you've done this if you find yourself counting sugar cones rather than sheep when you're trying to get to sleep!)

Here are some proven strategies for keeping the hunger pangs at bay:

- Tap into the power of H_2O—good, old-fashioned water! If you get into the habit of drinking a glass of water before and during your meals, you'll consume less food. (The reason is obvious: the water helps to fill you up. There's also growing evidence that your body burns calories more efficiently when its cells are fully hydrated.) If you're no great fan of water (or you can't imagine downing the requisite eight or more glasses per day), don't be afraid to reach for a glass of tomato juice instead. Not only will it help to fill your stomach—it's also packed with nutrients. And if you suspend your credibility a little, you can almost—I repeat almost—convince yourself that the creamy texture means that you're enjoying a deliciously decadent treat. (Hey, you've got to have a good imagination if you want to become an Incredible Shrinking Woman!)
- Eat bulky foods that will help to fill you up: everything from vegetables to baked beans to whole-

> ### Food for Thought
>
> Here's another good reason to hit the water cooler. According to Diane Irons, author of *The World's Best-Kept Diet Secrets*, your body burns 40 calories trying to bring each glass of ice-cold water up to body temperature.

The Skinny

Can't bear to part with your morning glass of orange juice? Dilute it with water or club soda. You'll get the same volume for half the calories.

grain breads. These foods take longer to digest so they leave you feeling full longer.

- Don't drink your calories when you can eat them instead. For the amount of calories you get in a single eight-ounce glass of orange juice, you could sit down and polish off two medium oranges.
- Reduce your "calories per minute" by choosing foods that take longer to eat. Not only are you likely to get more eating satisfaction from foods you can savour—you're also likely to eat less.

- Watch your intake of artificially sweetened products. One study showed that people who consume diet pop on a regular basis tend to feel hungrier than those who drink unsweetened or naturally sweet beverages.
- Don't skip meals or consume fewer than 300 to 400 calories at a meal. Starving yourself or serving yourself meagre rations doesn't speed up your weight loss. It merely increases the odds that you'll abandon your weight-loss program entirely.
- Stop viewing hunger signals as the enemy. Instead, recognize them for what they are: your body's signal that it wants good food. Since she started losing weight, Kathryn has learned to trust her hunger signals rather than be alarmed by them: "I try to let my appetite do its thing," she explains. "If I'm extra hungry one day, I figure there must be a good reason for it, like maybe I'm expending more energy or something. If I do eat more, I make sure that I'm eating more of the right things, like more fruits or more veggies. Sometimes I'll allow myself an extra snack in the afternoon if I need it. And if I know I've eaten a lot during the day, I tend to work harder at the gym that evening."

The Skinny

"I never let myself get hungry. When I started to lose weight, I brought in all kinds of low-fat, low-calorie snacks and had them around and ready to eat. I also drank tons of water."

— Dawnette, who is now within 10 pounds of her goal weight

(10) Learn to Differentiate Between Hunger and Cravings

Don't reach for food right away if you start feeling hungry. Instead, ask yourself if it's genuine hunger that you're feeling or just a powerful craving. "I try to distract myself for ten minutes," says Margaret. "Sometimes that helps. Also, drinking a big glass of water instead of eating can help."

It's also important to learn to tell the difference between thirst or fatigue and actual hunger. According to the obesity experts, we frequently confuse the need for a drink or a good night's sleep with the need for food.

(11) Come Up with a Game Plan for Handling Your Trigger Foods

We've all got our own trigger foods: foods that we can't seem to eat in moderation. According to Dr. Stephen Gullo, author of *Thin Tastes Better: Control Your Food Triggers Without Feeling Deprived*, trigger foods are less likely to be healthy foods like broccoli and carrots (how many people do you know who admit to having a problem with vegetables?) and more likely to be high-sugar, high-fat treats. He argues that most people are more likely to have problems with certain types of trigger foods than other types of foods: in other words, you might have a thing for sweet, creamy foods like chocolate and ice cream, or you might totally lose control when you're faced with salty foods like nuts or potato chips.

Here are some ways to manage your trigger foods:

- Come up with a list of your all-time favourite treats and then pick the one that you simply couldn't live without. Give yourself permission to have this item once during the week—assuming, of course, you actually want it.

  "For me, the biggest challenge was thinking I would never be able to have McDonald's or some other indulgent treat again," says Amy, who recently lost 67 pounds. "To cope with it, I taught myself to incorporate treats into my plan at least once a week (or even several times a week). This way, I never felt deprived. Of course, I lost the craving for super-sized fries and all that other greasy stuff pretty quickly, so my treats became less extravagant over time."

- Only buy single-serving sizes of your favourite foods. One study showed that you're likely to eat

Food for Thought

Here's further proof that men and women really are from different planets. According to a recent article in *Life* magazine, when men are depressed, they crave high-fat foods like pizza or hot dogs. Women, on the other hand, tend to crave chocolate.

The Skinny

"I have learned that no matter how motivated I am to succeed on my weight-loss program, I am prone to emotional eating. That's why I try not to have chocolate in the house, even for baking. If I do, I will go for that if my husband and I have argued or the kids are driving me up the wall."

— Elizabeth, who is currently trying to lose weight

The Skinny

Can't figure out how you're going to resist the urge to eat handfuls of cookie batter while you're doing your holiday baking? Pay a friend to do it for you. Not only will you be free of the temptation to lick the bowl, the spoon, and every other cooking utensil in sight— your house will also be free of the mouthwatering scent of freshly baked cookies.

44 percent more food if you buy these foods in multi-serving packages.

- Banish your favourite foods from home until you feel like you can regain control over them. If other members of the family have to indulge in the very types of delectables that you haven't got a hope of resisting, ask them to do their indulging elsewhere.

(12) Learn to Make Choices

Learn how to budget your food calories much as you budget your money. If you want to indulge in a high-fat dessert, go lighter on the entrée. Healthy eating—like life itself—is a matter of making choices.

(13) Be Portion Savvy

It's hard to imagine the number of weight-loss programs that have been sabotaged by something as apparently simple as portion control. Studies at St. Luke's-Roosevelt Hospital in New York City have shown that obese people tend to underestimate by more than 50% the number of calories that they consume. Rather than eating 1200 calories like they estimated they were, they were actually consuming upwards of 2000 calories per day. The lesson to be learned is obvious: when in doubt, measure.

The Skinny

"People who are successful at weight loss don't feel sorry for themselves. Their attitude is that it's worth it to give something up for what they get in return. If you want to lose weight but you also want to eat a lot of food, you'll have to choose one or the other. Ask yourself, 'Which one do I want more?'"

— Anne B. Fletcher, author of *Thin for Life*, quoted in *The Complete Idiot's Guide to Losing Weight*

(14) Trim, Don't Chop

Rather than going cold-turkey as you make the switch from high-fat to low-fat eating, wean yourself off fat gradually. Find ways to trim the fat from your favourite recipes rather than scrapping them in favour of something new.

Here are a few pointers:

- Experiment with new ways of cooking vegetables. Rather than sautéing them in oil, cook them in tomato juice, bouillon, or dry white wine. Don't be surprised if you have to up the quantity of liquid when you make the switch from oil: the tomato juice, bouillon, and wine will tend to evaporate more quickly while you're cooking.
- Reduce the amount of meat in your main dishes. Up the quantity of vegetables and cut back on the amount of meat when you're making chicken or beef stew, and try adding sautéed vegetables to your spaghetti sauce so that you won't need to throw in as much lean ground beef.

> **Food for Thought**
>
> Don't forget to factor in the extra calories that you add to packaged foods. That package of low-fat instant pudding may contain a measly 25 calories per serving, but the moment you add the skim milk, you triple the number of calories. (Guess you could say that the proof is in the pudding!)

- Replace high-fat cheeses in pasta dishes with lower-fat alternatives. You can tell how much fat is in a particular type of cheese by looking for the butterfat or milk fat ratings on dairy products. As a rule of thumb, you should aim for cheeses in the 7 to 15% BF or MF range. (Just a word of warning, in case you've never tasted a low-fat cheese in your life. Some low-fat cheeses are delicious. Others are unspeakably awful. I've had good luck buying low-fat Swiss and mozzarella cheese, but I've never found a low-fat cheddar that I could actually live with.)
- Use lower-calorie butter, margarine, and mayonnaise in sandwiches and other foods. Better yet, replace them with something else entirely, like mustard or a fat-free tahini spread.
- Replace some or all of the sour cream or cream cheese in your favourite recipes with puréed cottage cheese. Not only is it lower in fat content: it's also higher in protein content—something that can help to put your appetite on hold a little longer.
- If you're looking for something to replace that dollop of sour cream on a plate of nachos, try blending the sour cream with yogurt and gradually weaning yourself off your sour cream fix. (Note: While yogurt can double as sour cream when it comes to texture, it can't quite hold it's own in the taste department. If you decide to go this route, you'll probably want to slather on the salsa until your taste buds have a chance to fall in love with low-fat yogurt!)

- Replace some of the oil, shortening, butter, or margarine in cakes, cookies, and muffins with plain low-fat yogurt. (Note: You can't eliminate all the oil or you'll end up with baked goods with the texture of leather!)

Note: You can find plenty of great tips on low-fat cooking in such five-star cookbooks as *Tailoring Your Tastes* by Linda Omichinski and Heather Wiebe Hildebrand, and *Looneyspoons* or *Crazy Plates* by Janet and Greta Podleski, all of which get a regular workout in my kitchen. You can also find some fabulous low-fat recipes in Appendix F.

(15) Master the Art of Dining Out

You can't avoid eating out forever—nor would you want to! One of the best ways to give yourself a nice pick-me-up during the first week of your new weight-loss program is to treat yourself to a healthy dinner out.

Here are some tips on sticking to your weight-loss program while you're dining out:

- Look for a restaurant that features poached, steamed, broiled, boiled, or grilled entrées rather than their fried or deep-fried counterparts.
- Avoid restaurants that feature all-you-can-eat buffets—unless, of course, you're lucky enough to stumble across one with an all-you-can-eat lettuce and bean sprouts buffet. (Relax, I'm just kidding.) Most buffets are packed with high-fat foods like macaroni salads, fried chicken, and meatloaf that's positively swimming in gravy. That, of course, is the healthy stuff—at least compared to what you'll find in the dessert lineup. You'll encounter coconut cream pies, butter tarts, marshmallow-and-Jell-O salads and other high-fat holdovers from the 1950s.
- Ask for a glass of water the moment you're seated at your table. It'll help to fill you up while you decide what you want to order for dinner.
- Have a clear soup or a large green salad before your dinner arrives. It'll take the edge of your appetite before your entrée arrives.
- Request that all salad dressings, gravies, and sauces be served on the side. That way, you'll be able to control the amount that ends up on your food.

The Skinny

Don't stand next to the food table when you're at a party. It's too easy to nibble non-stop. Position yourself on the other side of the room and hold your drink in the wrong hand. That way, you'll be less adept at helping yourself to the hors d'oeuvres that end up making their way around the room.

- If your entrée is huge, ask the waiter to split it in half. That way, you can take the other half of your meal home to enjoy for lunch the next day.
- Can't find a suitable entrée? Order two appetizers instead. Team up a large green salad and a bowl of black bean soup and you'll have a dinner that's fit for a queen.
- Watch your alcohol consumption. Alcohol both increases your appetite and decreases your willpower. It's no wonder that studies have shown that people who drink alcoholic beverages tend to consume an average of 200 additional calories during the subsequent 24 hours.

(16) Know When to Shut Your Mouth—Literally

One of the most difficult times of the day for anyone who is trying to lose weight is the evening. Once dinner is finished, you're faced with a 12-hour wait until your next meal. Is it any wonder that so many of us switch into munchie mode?

Here are some tips on coping with the mid-evening munchies:

- Get out of the kitchen. You're more likely to obsess about food if it's staring you right in the face. Out of sight, out of hand.
- Brush and floss your teeth after dinner. You're less likely to reach for a mid-evening snack if you know you've got to go to all the bother of cleaning them again.
- Have a firm policy when it comes to night-time snacking as well as a fall-back position. While you might choose to avoid night-time snacking most of the time, you might want to allow yourself a mid-evening snack if you're genuinely ravenous. (Note: The mid-evening munchies can strike if you've gone too light on eating during the day or if you've become so zealous about trimming the fat content from your evening meal that you end up eliminating a lot of the protein content at the same time.)

The Skinny

Don't forget to plan ahead when you're travelling. You're less likely to succumb to temptation if you keep these tips in mind:

- Bring your own snacks. It'll be easier to say no to the free peanuts that are offered to you by the flight attendant or the goodies that are waiting in the mini-bar in your hotel room if you know you've got a healthy snack that you can eat instead.
- Pack your running shoes in your carry-on luggage. That way, if you get hit with an unexpected flight delay, you can go for a walk rather than hitting the airport cafeteria.
- If someone's making your travel arrangements for you, let them know that you're trying to lose weight. That way, they can try to find you a hotel that boasts both top-notch exercise facilities and a restaurant that dishes up healthy meals.

Food for Thought

Nursing mothers have an advantage when it comes to losing weight. A woman typically burns an extra 500 to 700 calories per day while she's breastfeeding a baby. What's more, these women are able to draw upon that oh-so-stubborn fat on their thighs and buttocks—fat that's been stashed away for this very purpose! This can have a dramatic affect on weight-loss efforts: a typical woman's thighs account for approximately 25 percent of her body weight.

• If all else fails, go to bed early. You won't consume any calories while you're sleeping—unless, of course, you happen to be a sleepwalker!

(17) Put Your Best Foot Forward

Give your metabolism a boost by getting active right from the very start of your weight-loss program. Not only will exercising help you to build muscle—something that will increase the number of calories that your body burns on a day-to-day basis—you'll also be able to counter the metabolic drop that often occurs when you start a weight-loss program.

Now that I've given you the lowdown on some tricks of the trade that should help you to weather the highs and lows of the critical first week, it's time to focus on another aspect of weight control: your relationship with the scale!

To Weigh or Not to Weigh?

"Sometimes I love it; sometimes I hate it," says Kathryn, who recently lost 70 pounds. "Sometimes I'm damned scared of it! It vindicates me and it punishes me. I feel all sorts of emotions about that dastardly scale!"

Are you having a love-hate relationship with your bathroom scale? If you are, you're certainly in good company. Most of the women I know could fill a therapy session or two talking about nothing more than that five-pound hunk of metal!

In fact, I think Heather (one of the women I interviewed for this book) is one of the few women I know who has managed to put the scale in its place. She keeps hers in the garage! Not only is the floor more level out there than in the house—banishing it to the great outdoors prevents the scale from driving her crazy on a day-to-day or hour-to-hour basis. I don't know about you, but I think Heather's a genius. I mean, you're less likely to get hung up about weighing yourself in the nude each morning if you have to trek out to the garage in order to do so. (That wouldn't exactly be a lot of fun in the middle of February!) Still, there's always a downside to consider: imagine what would happen if some neighbour with an el cheapo garage door opener caused *your* garage door to go flying up at the exact moment you dropped your towel and stepped on the scale!

As you can see, we've got plenty to talk about in this chapter: how often you should weigh yourself, why the scale can be your worst enemy, and why it's important to find other ways than weighing yourself to measure your weight-loss success.

The Weighing Game

How often should you weigh yourself? Once a day? Once a week? Once a month? Never? Not even the experts have been able to come up with a definitive answer to this particular question. Some suggest that you throw away your scale altogether, while others argue that weighing yourself periodically is a good way to monitor your weight-loss success.

Dr. Debra Waterhouse, author of *Outsmarting the Female Fat Cell*, encourages women to get rid of their scales entirely: "I don't even have a scale in my office," she writes. "When clients come in for their first appointment, they quickly scan the room and ask, 'OK, where's the scale? In the closet?' When I tell them that I don't have one, they are surprised and sometimes a little perturbed: 'You mean I fasted all day yesterday for nothing?'... Do yourself a favor and throw away the scale or put it in the garage—at least for the next three months."

Dr. Miriam Nelson, author of *Strong Women Stay Slim*, agrees that the scale can be a source of frustration for many women, but notes that others find it to be a valuable tool. That's why she suggests that each woman make up her own mind about the frequency of weigh-ins: "In my experience, some women do just fine with daily weighing. They're prepared for variations and can focus on long-term trends. Others avoid the scale and track their progress in other ways. That's okay too. Figure out which approach works best for you."

Elizabeth is one of those women who likes to keep tabs on her weight on a regular basis. She has discovered that weighing herself twice a day—morning and night—helps to keep her focused on her weight-loss program: "I don't think it's necessary [to weigh myself that often], but I like to know whether or not I'm actually losing."

Margaret has found that weighing herself on a much less regular basis is a better solution for her: "I usually weigh myself about once a week or not at all. I don't always find that the scale reflects how I feel about how I'm doing. For example, if I think I'm doing great and I weigh myself and I haven't lost anything, I can get discouraged."

Here are some factors to consider when you're trying to decide how often to hop on the scale:

- **Are you a perfectionist?** If you are, you might find it hard to cope with a disappointing result on the scale. You might choose to weigh yourself somewhere other than at home (so you won't be tempted to weigh yourself a dozen times a day and drive yourself crazy in the process!) or find ways other than weighing yourself to track your weight loss.

- **Are you an emotional eater**? Are you likely to turn to the refrigerator for solace if the scale reveals a disappointing result, even if you know that you've been eating sensibly and exercising regularly?
- **Will the scale help to keep you honest or will it encourage you to cheat**? Will you feel more committed than ever to your weight-loss program

if the scale shows a loss or will you decide that you deserve to treat yourself to a massive slab of cheesecake because you've been doing so well?

Answering these questions should help you to decide whether you'd be better off weighing yourself on a daily basis or taking a sledgehammer to the temperamental metal contraption on your bathroom floor.

Why the Scale Can Be Your Worst Enemy

Margaret isn't the only one who lets the number on the scale control her mood. Krista—who has lost 50 pounds over the past year—finds it very hard to deal with the disappointment that she feels when the scale shows a gain rather than a loss: "If I gain two pounds, it's like the end of the world for me," she admits. "I feel like it is going to take me forever to lose weight and that my efforts are useless. I have had to ask myself how much two pounds matters when I get mad at the scales for showing a gain. Perfectionism is a huge hindrance for me in the scale department. I let the scale control my moods."

Jill—who is halfway to her goal of losing 120 pounds—has found that a disappointing result on the scale can cause her to become less committed to her weight-loss program: "I feel like the scale sabotages my weight-loss plans sometimes," she confesses. "If I don't see a good drop in weight after some apocalyp-

The Skinny

"Weighing myself can be an advantage when the scale shows a loss. It helps to motivate me to keep up the good work. On the other hand, when the scale shows a gain, it can be very discouraging or depressing even."

— Margaret, who is currently trying to lose weight

The Skinny

"I have become obsessive about the numbers—especially weighing myself every day. The number on the scale can have an unrealistic impact on my mood: if I'm down two pounds, I'm happy; if I'm up two pounds, I'm depressed. Those mood swings based on the number on the scale can wreak havoc on my motivation for the day."

— Jill, who is halfway to her goal of losing 120 pounds

The Skinny

"Don't let that blasted scale discourage you. There are times when your weight is up or down by a pound or two in a matter of three days and it doesn't mean you're eating more or less than you should, and it isn't necessarily affected by exercise either. Don't let the fluctuations affect your eating or exercise habits. Just keep chugging along and you will have weight-loss success. If you keep your 'weigh days' down to once a week, you'll feel better about your overall success."

— Kathryn, who recently lost 70 pounds

tic week when I've been absolutely perfect and exercised like a triathlete, then I feel defeated and may choose to eat a bit more and exercise a bit less the following week."

Other Ways to Measure Your Success

If you're relying on the scale as the sole measure of your weight-loss success, you're setting yourself up for disappointment.

For one thing, your standard Heinz 57 bathroom scale tends to be anything but accurate. Consider the $50 model in my bathroom upstairs. If I hop on and off the scale three different times, I'm guaranteed to get three different results, and it's not unusual for there to be a couple of pounds difference between the highest and lowest reading on the scale.

But even if your scale is one of those rare beasts that can be counted on to give you the same result more than once, it could still be telling you half-truths. You see, the scale isn't capable of telling you how much of your body weight is made up of fat and how much is made up of bone and muscle weight—nor is it able to pinpoint whether a two-pound weight gain is due to PMS or the bag of Doritos you ate on the weekend. (This is a point we discussed at length back in Chapter 1, "The Skinny on Being Fat," but one that certainly warrants repeating.) Unless you enjoy driving yourself crazy, it's a good idea to find other ways to measure your success, whether or not you decide to ditch your scale.

Here are a few ideas:

- **Reach for a tape measure rather than turning to the bathroom scale for answers.** Sometimes your weight comes off in inches rather than pounds. This is particularly likely to be the case if you're exercising, since adding muscle can actually cause your weight to go up.

The Skinny

"Just think of the scale as one of the many tools available to you in your weight-loss efforts. It's not the be-all and end-all. If you are going to use the scale regularly, use it at the same time of the day on the same day of the week, if possible. Your weight can vary tremendously from hour to hour and day to day."

— Margaret, who is currently trying to lose weight

- **Ask yourself if you feel any thinner.** Does your stomach feel smaller? Do your arms feel firmer? Sometimes these subtle cues from your body can tell you a whole lot more about the success of your weight-loss program than any sweet nothing whispered in your ear by a talking scale!

- **Consider whether your clothes are fitting you any differently.** One of the first clues that my body gave me that I was losing weight and building muscle was the way my shirt sleeves felt on my upper arms. Rather than feeling like blood pressure cuffs (a sensation I'd become all too accustomed to!), the fabric actually hung loosely around my biceps. (Take a bow, nautilus machines!)

- **Look for other evidence that you've lost weight.** Do the chairs suddenly seem to have more room? Is your seat belt looser when you're travelling by car or by air? These are other important indications that the weight is coming off.

- **Focus on your overall fitness level rather than the number on the scale.** Rather than fixating on how much you've lost, think of what you've gained! If you've been eating properly and exercising regularly, you may have experienced a significant improvement in your overall fitness level—something that is far more worthy of a celebration than any number on the scale.

Now that we've talked about where the scale does—or doesn't—fit into your weight-loss program, let's move on to another important topic: the importance of staying motivated.

The Skinny

"The scale only provides a snapshot of a moment in time, and so much can effect that: where you're at in your menstrual cycle, the humidity, whether you've been exercising a lot, and so on. Just keep to your program because if you do, sooner or later you'll see the number you want on the scale."

— Susan, who is currently trying to lose weight

The Skinny

Understand your own personal weight-loss patterns. That way, you'll be less tempted to throw in the towel if the scale starts moving in the wrong direction. Consider what Amy—a veteran of the Battle of the Bulge—has to say about the importance of tracking your own weight-loss patterns: "I've found that I consistently gain weight or maintain my weight right before my period and right before ovulation. Understanding this cycle helped me not to feel frustrated during the weeks when I gained or when I maintained my weight even though I was being really 'good'."

9

Avoiding the Five Biggest Motivation Zappers

The Skinny

"I agree there is a honeymoon period. However, just like any good marriage, you learn to adapt after the honeymoon if you want to be successful."

— Barb, who has lost over 100 pounds over the past year

The first few weeks of a weight-loss program aren't unlike the first few weeks of married life: you're so thrilled by your "new life" that you can't help but see the world through rose-coloured glasses. At some point, however, the glasses come off and you begin to notice little things about your weight-loss program (or your beloved!) that begin to drive you crazy. (Your weight-loss program may not leave its socks next to the laundry hamper or start burping at the dinner table, but it can do a lot of equally annoying things. Trust me!)

In this chapter we're going to talk about what you can do to stay motivated once the honeymoon is officially over. We'll zero in on the five biggest motivation zappers and then we'll talk about ways to get back on the weight-loss wagon once you fall (or get thrown) off.

What to Do Once the Honeymoon's Over

It would be a lot easier to cope with the end of the honeymoon stage if you were able to predict in advance how long it might last. You could mark the date on your calendar and make a mental note to avoid driving past any Baskin Robbins outlets on your way home from work. Unfortunately, most of us aren't able to predict in advance when the honeymoon is going to come to an end and we're going to wake up and realize that weight loss (like marriage!) isn't always fun.

Tammie (who is currently losing weight) found that her honeymoon stage lasted for about two months. At that point, she abandoned some of her healthy eating habits: "I started to feel like since I was losing at a good pace, I could go ahead and eat some of the foods I had been avoiding. Big mistake! I gained!"

Jill—who is now halfway to her goal of losing 120 pounds—finds that she's constantly moving in and out of a honeymoon-like state: "I think I fluctuate between the honeymoon stage and the divorce stage all the time with my weight-loss program," she explains. "Some weeks I am incredibly motivated: I will cook for the week, plan my exercise, go shopping for healthy foods, and so on. Other weeks, I can barely open up a can of soup without cursing the fat on my body. For me, the motivation is on a continuum: some days, I'm way over on the highly motivated side; other days I'm on the 'let's drink a beer and eat a corn dog' side. The important thing for me is to try to stay in the middle most of the time and know that when I drift over to one side occasionally, to remember that the other side is going to be visited soon, too."

Shari feels that the honeymoon stage isn't necessarily a good thing for her: she feels more comfortable once reality sets in: "I'm a compulsive/obsessive eater, so the honeymoon stage never lasts long," she explains. "On the flip side, it always comes back around. My struggle, actually, is not to have any honeymoon stages. These are just artificial highs that plummet into almost insurmountable lows. I am striving for evenness in my thinking."

The Five Biggest Motivation Zappers

Wondering what causes weight-loss programs to go off the tracks? I've talked to a lot of women about this topic and I've concluded that there are five key reasons why women who have been successfully losing weight suddenly decide to throw in the towel.

(1) Impatience

As I stated earlier in this book, I was born without the gene for patience. When I embark on a weight-loss program, I want to see dramatic results right away. When I don't (mainly because I'm unwilling to sabotage my long-term success by trying

The Skinny

"I lose motivation if I don't see fast results. I find it hard to 'diet'—to be regimented, to exercise regularly. If I don't see results, I get resentful and I cave."

— Margaret, who is currently trying to lose weight

the hottest fad diet du jour) I tend to get discouraged and to start questioning whether it's actually worth the effort to stick with my weight-loss program.

In the past, Shari also found it hard to wait for the needle on the scale to start moving in the right direction. Over the past year, however, she's started to learn to be patient with herself—something that has helped to contribute to her success: "The biggest thing for me has been recognizing that it took me 43 years to get this way and that, with all my heart, I want the extra weight gone forever. The rate at which I lose weight no longer has any meaning for me. I am focused on progress in overcoming my eating disorder and I know that weight loss will eventually result. Each day that I can make progress in gaining control is a little miracle for me."

(2) Boredom

Does the mere thought of your weight-loss program make you break out in yawns? You could be about to fall prey to one of the biggest motivation zappers of all—boredom!

The Skinny

"Don't look at the big picture. If you look at all the weight you have to lose, it'll seem like so much that you'll be afraid to try. If you set small goals for yourself, like wanting to lose five pounds in two months, you'll be more successful. Even a small weight loss during that period can be enough to motivate you to keep going."

— Kathryn, who recently lost 70 pounds

Susan has discovered that boredom is a real problem for her when she's trying to lose weight: "Routine works best for me in the beginning. For about the first four or five weeks, I do exactly the same exercises in the exact same places and would gladly eat the same meals if necessary. But suddenly—and I mean suddenly—I will get very bored. This is the crucial point: I must either be prepared to make some changes to my routine or I will fail and return to my old nasty habits."

Kathryn has also discovered that an ounce of prevention is worth a pound of cure—at least when it comes to boredom: "I'm always looking for new low-fat recipes and trying new foods. Same with exercise. I change my exercise routine every two or three months. Right now, I'm jogging and weight training.

I'm getting ready to start learning tennis and I plan to take an aerobics class in a few weeks."

③ Failing to Meet Your Own Needs

One of the most effective ways of sabotaging your weight-loss success is to stop taking care of yourself. This past month, I got so busy working on book projects that I hardly managed to make it to the gym at all. Add to that the fact that I had sick kids, Christmas shopping, and a million-and-one-other crises to contend with and it's not difficult to figure out why my weight loss ground to a complete and utter halt. For the first time since I started losing weight eight months ago, I didn't even manage to lose a single ounce.

I now realize that I have sabotaged my weight-loss success over the years by allowing myself to get too busy. I've discovered (mainly by performing weight gain postmortems!) that if I don't have time to do all the things that help me lose weight—hitting the gym on a regular basis, shopping for healthy foods, making healthy meals, and spending a few moments each day focusing on my weight-loss goals—it's easy for me to throw in the towel.

To make matters worse, I've discovered that I tend to turn to food for comfort at times like these. Clearly, there's a loose wire in my brain that causes my signals to get a little scrambled: time and time again, I've fallen into the trap of convincing myself that a handful of licorice all-sorts is a good substitute for rest, relaxation, exercise, and healthy foods—all the things my body actually needs!

I know that the key to getting my weight-loss program on track again is to do the one thing that seems most difficult for me to do: dumping some of my work and family commitments and setting aside more time for myself. Unless I'm content to tread water indefinitely at a decidedly unsvelte 189 pounds, it's time for me to get with the program again.

④ Losing Your Focus

Another effective way to ensure that your weight-loss dreams go up in smoke is to allow yourself to lose sight of why you ever wanted to lose weight in the first place. After all, if you've lost enough weight that you're no longer huffing and puffing each time you run up a flight or stairs and you're short a chin or two when you look in the mirror, you might be just as content to stay where you are than to continue losing weight.

There's nothing wrong with waving the weight-loss white flag at this point, of course—deciding to put the brakes on your weight-loss efforts and focus on maintaining your loss, at least for now. Frankly, that's a far saner alternative than forcing yourself to stick with a weight-loss program that your heart is no longer in. But if you do decide that you're not happy with the weight you've achieved—that you do want to drop some additional pounds—then you need to find a way to focus on your weight-loss goals once again.

Amy—who recently lost 67 pounds—discovered that it helped her to have something else to focus on in addition to her weight-loss goals: training for a marathon. "I didn't run in order to lose weight. I ran because I had to keep my mileage up in order to complete the race. Having the race to focus on allowed me to keep my spirits up during weeks when my losses weren't spectacular. It also helped to keep me motivated after the initial excitement of losing weight."

(5) Letting Success Go to Your Head

Success is a good thing, right? Yes and no. Believe it or not, success can actually sabotage your weight-loss efforts. As the pounds begin to come off and people around you start telling you how great you're looking, it's easy to let that initial success go to your head. Suddenly, it doesn't seem nearly so important to continue to lose weight: after all, you're already getting the chance to enjoy the compliments and other perks. In fact, there's so much to say about the joys and perils of success that I've devoted the final chapter of the book to this particular topic. (Don't touch that dial!)

How to Get Back on the Weight-Loss Wagon Once You've Fallen Off

In a perfect world, no one would ever fall off the weight-loss wagon. We'd all have time to exercise the requisite three to five times per week, to hit the grocery store on a regular basis, and to whip up mouthwatering meals that could satisfy even the most discriminating gourmet. Well, I don't know about you, but my day-to-day life generally falls a little short of perfection, something that helps to explain why my motivation tends to waver from time to time.

And then, of course, there's the fact that I'm still using my training wheels when it comes to living a healthy lifestyle. I've got 35 years of so-so eating and exercise habits (frankly, I'm being a little generous with that assessment!) and less than a year of healthy eating to my credit. This means that it's still all-too-easy for me to fall back into an old habit without even realizing that I'm doing so.

> ## The Skinny
>
> "Everyone slips now and then. Don't be self-critical if that happens. Focus on all the positive things you've been able to accomplish. If you could do all this, you can certainly get back on track."
>
> — Miriam Nelson, *Strong Women Stay Slim*

Let me give you a non-food example of how powerful this "programming" can be. I have gotten into the habit of hanging up my coat in the front hall closet the moment I walk through the front door at home. It's something that's so automatic that I hardly even think about it. But when I go to visit my parents, I automatically hang my coat on the doorknob—a habit of mine that they've spent a good twenty years trying to break! If it's this easy for me to slip pack into my old ways when it comes to being a slob—something I'm not particularly emotionally attached to, despite what my mother might tell you!—imagine how much easier it is for me to fall back into my old eating habits from time to time.

As you can see, it's hardly surprising at all that we tend to fall off the weight-loss wagon from time to time. Since most of us find it difficult to avoid these spills altogether, we need to know how to prevent a momentary accident from turning into a permanent stopover! Here are some proven strategies for getting your weight-loss program back on track when you've committed the mortal sin of (gasp!) being human:

- **Put on the brakes.** The sooner you can stop yourself from engaging in out-of-control eating, the less damage you'll do. The best solution of all, of course, is to head off a bout of overeating before it occurs—perhaps by reaching out for support from a friend who understands what it's like to wrestle with the Eating Monster or by making it harder for yourself to lose control. (If a particular food is calling your name, you might want to go for a walk or throw it in the garbage can fast.) If you can't prevent the overeating from occurring in the first place, at least admit to yourself that it's happened and then put on the brakes.

The Skinny

"With most compulsive eaters, the moment of awakening comes long after the moment of truth—that split second when we tell ourselves The Big Lie. 'Just one bite.' 'Oh, this is nothing: I've been good all day.' 'I deserve it.' 'It's a special occasion.' 'Well, I can't just go hungry, can I?' 'This is all that's available.' … The most important thing is that you take a breath, take a step back (literally, step away from the food!), and ask yourself, 'Is this taking me one step closer to my goal or one step further away from my goal? Don't lie to yourself. (If you do lie to yourself, then don't believe the lie!) Then do whatever it takes to walk away."

— Shari, who has lost 13 pounds toward her goal of a 53-pound weight loss

The Skinny

"I've learned not to wallow in a setback or a failure. If I eat something I shouldn't, I don't let it get too far beyond that one incident. I don't continue to eat poorly the next day. I just move on and continue with my program."

— Margaret, who is currently trying to lose weight

• **Keep your perspective.** If you're starting to obsess about what an awful person you are because you happened to hoover an entire box of Timbits, let me remind you that you're not exactly a gun-toting criminal. You didn't rob a bank, cheat a little old lady out of her retirement savings, or steal a tricycle from a little kid. You simply fell off your weight-loss program.

• **Resist the temptation to "punish" yourself.** We have a funny way of punishing ourselves when we fall of the weight-loss wagon, don't we? I mean we try to teach ourselves a lesson by shovelling in more food! (I don't know about you, but I don't see the logic here myself. Not that I haven't been guilty of doing just that on more occasions that I'd be prepared to admit, mind you: it's just that it doesn't make any sense!) This was certainly Jill's pattern in the past—a pattern that she's managed to break in her current weight-loss program: "I used to be fanatical about diets I was on," she explains. "Now I'm more mellow. I stay on track as best I can, but if I put something in my mouth that's high-calorie, it doesn't ruin my day. Years ago, if I ate anything that wasn't 'on the program,' I would chastise myself by eating ice cream for the rest of the day (or week, depending on my offence)."

• **Focus on how far you've come.** A day—or even a week—of out-of-control eating doesn't automatically erase all the hard work you've put into your program. Even if you do manage to gain a pound or two, you've already proven to yourself that you've got the necessary skills to shed those pounds again. Krista—a natural-born perfectionist—is slowly but surely learning to see the weight-loss glass as 90% full rather than 10% empty: "I still fail, but I am beginning to understand that life is about falling down and getting back up again—about starting over, but not all the way back to square one. I am okay with three steps forward and one step back."

- **Forgive yourself and move on.** Don't fall into the trap of letting one bad day—or even one bad week—short-circuit your entire weight-loss program. When I'm having a hard time forgiving myself for "blowing it," I remind myself that I've still got a weight loss "batting average" that could put any major league baseball player to shame: I figure I'm batting about .900!

- **Resist the urge to starve yourself to make up for the weight-loss faux pas.** It's tempting to cut back your food intake dramatically in order to make up for your temporary digression, but it's not a good idea. Geneen Roth explains why in her book *When You Eat at the Refrigerator, Pull Up a Chair:* "Starving yourself after overeating only leads to another cycle of overeating and starving yourself. It doesn't lead to weight loss, health, well-being, or balanced energy. It also makes you feel like a lunatic, since hunger is a survival mechanism. You need to eat to live. When you deny your hunger, even the day after you've consumed thousands of calories, you are also denying the life force that keeps you alive."

How to "Re-motivate" Yourself

You spent a lot of time motivating yourself at the start of your weight-loss program. An excellent way to get back on track when you've fallen off the wagon is to spend some time "re-motivating" yourself.

Here are some proven strategies for recharging your motivation batteries:

The Skinny

"I like things to be right and structured. When things get out of hand and I don't attend to the matter immediately, then they appear to be unfixable and I give up and wallow in the abyss. That happens to me with housecleaning, weight loss, and every other aspect of my life. This time, I am trying to set smaller goals. I am trying not to think about what I should achieve by the end of the week. Instead, I set half-day goals so that things don't get out of hand. The big picture is still in my mind, but that is still about 95 pounds away, so I set the small goals to get there."

— Susan, who is currently trying to lose weight

The Skinny

"I just remember to keep putting one foot in front of the other, and I'm gentle with myself. Weight loss, like life, goes in cycles. Some days are better than others; some periods are better than others. If you do your best and keep moving forward, even when that forward motion is slower than you'd prefer at times, you always get where you're going."

— Jenna, who recently lost 90 pounds

The Skinny

"I try on clothes that make me feel good—clothes that I couldn't fit into a month ago. I look at old pictures versus new pictures of myself and see what a difference there is. It makes me feel good, like it's all been worthwhile. That keeps me from doing anything drastic to jeopardize the weight loss."

— Kathryn, who recently lost 70 pounds

- **Confront the naked truth.** Take off your clothes and stand in front of your mirror. Focus on how much progress you've made in losing weight to date and how much more weight you hope to lose. If you're not into nude meditation, you might want to try Tammie's approach instead: "I try on clothing that never would have fit me six months ago and think about where I will be next summer, next Christmas, and so on, if I don't dive into that sea of calories."
- **Get a mental picture of yourself at a slimmer weight.** It's no wonder that athletes use positive visualization to take themselves across the finish line. This is pretty powerful stuff! "Although I had difficulty with it at first, I strongly believe that visualization is helping me tremendously," says Susan. "I see myself at my goal. I see what I am wearing. I smell the air. I feel the breeze on my body. I hear the ocean. I am aware of my surroundings. I feel myself being healthy and happy. I practise this as often as I can during the day." Krista agrees that positive visualization can make a huge difference: "I think about how I am going to feel when I get to my goal: the clothes I will wear and the way that I will be able to do things and not just sit on the sidelines."
- **Remind yourself of all the other benefits of losing weight.** Make a list (mental or on paper) of all the benefits to losing weight: being able to run across a parking lot without wondering if you're going to collapse, having more energy to do things you want to do, and feeling more comfortable with your body. (If you're running short of ideas, be sure to flip back to Chapter 1, "The Skinny on Being Fat.")
- **Consider what might happen if you were to throw in the towel at this point.** If thinking positively won't motivate you, you might have to scare yourself into getting back on track. This is what Susan does if she's having a hard time staying on

The Skinny

"You have to think positively. You have to envision yourself at your goal each and every day when you're trying to lose weight—especially if you have more than thirty pounds to lose, or even 70 or more pounds to lose, like I did. It doesn't happen very quickly, so if you don't think positively, you can get easily discouraged and give up."

— Kathryn, who recently lost 70 pounds

track with her weight-loss program: "I think I'm motivated by the fact that I'm now 41 and am starting to feel aches and pains that I never felt before and I don't want to be incapacitated any more than I already am. Maybe it's because there was so much I wanted to do in my life like sky diving, rock climbing, and running marathons, but now time may not allow it. Maybe it's that I haven't felt sexy in a long while. So I guess that what keeps me motivated is fear: Fear of being unhealthy, ugly, sad, and unfulfilled for the rest of my life."

- **Realize that success begets success.** Sometimes the best thing you can do to get your weight-loss program back on track is to experience some more success. That technique certainly works for Elizabeth: "If I've started losing again and can see a difference, that's usually enough to spur me on. I can almost see my halo when I stick to my weight-loss plan!"

Want to hear even more about success? (Frankly, I can't blame you! All this talk about falling off the wagon has been kind of a downer.) Well, guess what? You're in luck. That's exactly what we're going to be talking about in the next and final chapter of this book.

The Skinny

"My motivation this time is to break free of the chains that obesity has placed on me. Whether those chains are physical (because I just can't do things I like), emotional (because of fear of what others will say, or of hurting myself), or social (because being fat limits opportunity), there are things I still want to do in life that I am not doing. My motivation is to live life to the fullest and to stop apologizing for who I am."

— Catherine, who is currently losing weight

The Skinny

"I look at old 'fat' pictures of myself. I think about how hard it was to climb stairs when I was overweight and out of shape. I dig down deep into myself to find my 'inner athlete' who enjoys the shape she's in and wants to keep eating right and exercising to improve that shape even more. It helps me to just take a moment and evaluate why I'm feeling unmotivated: what's the problem that's keeping me from staying on track? I think about how wonderful it feels to have lost the weight and how horrible it would be to gain it back."

— Kathryn, who recently lost 70 pounds

The Sweet Taste of Success

Once upon a time, there was a beautiful princess who was about 100 pounds overweight. She started eating healthy foods, exercising regularly, and—most important of all—she kicked her rather disgusting habit of kissing every frog who came along. After months of following the trendy diet plan popularized by those pint-sized weight-loss gurus the Seven Dwarfs, she finally managed to reach her goal weight. She might have lived happily ever after if it weren't for a bit of bad luck: instead of reaching for the slab of cheesecake that she found in the middle of the woods, she took the more virtuous route and ate the poisonous apple. As luck would have it, the prince who happened by didn't like skinny women and couldn't bear the thought of kissing her. That was the end of the beautiful princess.

Most of us are used to reading stories with happy endings. We find it more than a little disconcerting when people don't get too live "happily ever after"—particularly if they've followed the "rules" by losing weight! (After all, don't thin thighs and a tight butt practically guarantee you a happy ending? That's the line I've been fed all these years.)

As much as you might like to believe that losing weight will guarantee you a happy ending in all areas of your life—that your problems will disappear along with the extra pounds, thanks to some new fat-blocking magic wand—that's simply not the case. As any veteran "loser" can tell you, the weight-loss world tends to be distinctly un-fairytale-like. (Let's see if my editors allow me to keep that particular word!) In fact, if I were you, the only lesson I'd take away from the whole Snow White story is the importance of eating fresh produce. After all, if that apple had been fresh-picked, she could have saved herself a whole lot of grief.

As you may have gathered by now, the subject of this final chapter is happy versus unhappy endings: in other words, the joys and perils of success. Once we've talked about what success really means, we're going to talk about the $10 000 question: what it takes to maintain your weight loss over the long term.

The Joys of Success

It's not hard to sit down and write a list of all the reasons to feel joyful about losing weight. In fact, that's exactly what Kathryn did after she finished losing 70 pounds: she jotted down ten reasons she was happy about losing weight—everything from being able to take stairs two at a time "without getting even a little winded" to "liking what I see when I look in the mirror—from any angle."

While Kathryn had tried to lose weight in the past, something really clicked for her during her most recent weight-loss attempt: "I was more dedicated this time. I was a woman on a mission. I guess I was just fed up with being overweight. I knew how I wanted to look and I decided to do anything and everything I could to look that way and feel that way, too. I wanted to feel healthier."

Kathryn is not the first to admit that losing weight is hard work, but she's convinced that the sacrifices were worth it: "Success to me means feeling good about the way I look and my health in general. Losing weight gave me something incredibly valuable: confidence in myself. I have increased self-esteem and feel as

The Skinny

"I believe that you have to find a certain peace within yourself to be ready to go on a weight-loss program. It's an entirely personal choice. This choice cannot be made because someone else wants you to lose weight or you feel you have to because of outside influences. It has to be for you and only you. I started losing weight because I wanted to get back in touch with the me I always imagined I could be. Sure, that's partly cosmetic—wanting to look more attractive—but it's also about feeling good about myself. And after losing 70 pounds, I am more confident. I feel like a strong, centred woman. Now that I've lost this weight, I feel like I can do anything. Growing up, I was a very insecure child and I had a horrible body image. Now, I have a much better body image and, like I said, I feel much more confident."

— Kathryn, who recently lost 70 pounds

Food for Thought

"Sometimes weight loss stops when you're still heavier than you want to be. You try cutting back on food, but skimpier rations leave you hungry. Adding aerobic exercise isn't appealing either—you're already working out five days a week, for a total of five hours. This situation calls for reassessment of your weight-loss goals."

— Miriam Nelson, *Strong Women Stay Slim*

if there is increased purpose to my life—all from just losing weight. This new me can talk better, walk better, feel better, act better. It's all better."

Do-It-Yourself Success

Not every woman who loses weight defines success as reaching her "ideal" weight, of course. In fact, every woman has a very personal definition of what weight-loss success means to her.

Some women, like Shari, measure success in terms of their ability to kick a lifetime of compulsive eating habits, regardless of what number shows up on the scale. "If I have learned one thing in my determination to end my obsession with eating, it is that the problem, the solution, and all definitions of success in between are highly individual," she insists. "Success for me is being free of what I call the Monster—the guy in my head who exhorts me to eat and can't rest when there's food nearby."

Others—like Amy—are happy to stabilize at a weight that's a little higher than their "ideal" because they feel that the higher weight is a weight that they have at least a fighting chance of being able to maintain. "How I feel and what I can accomplish are more important than the number inside my jeans. For me, the right weight is the one that I feel good at, but also don't have to constantly monitor my food intake and energy output to maintain. At one point, I was 29 pounds lighter than my goal weight, and every day was a struggle just to stay at that weight. I couldn't treat myself at even one meal without paying for it at the scale. To me, that's not living. To have a body like that—even though it looked great—was not worth the sacrifice. Now I'm happy with a weight that's in a healthy BMI range, that allows me to do sports and other daily activities at a comfortable pace, and that allows me to shop in a normal clothing store."

Some women are surprised to find themselves feeling successful relatively early on in their weight-loss journeys: "It is the strangest thing," Susan

The Skinny

"Success feels like I am the most powerful person around. It feels like the ball and chain have been made lighter and that some day they will be removed completely. It feels like the deepest and cleanest breath of fresh air."

— Susan, who has lost 30 pounds toward her goal of losing 110 pounds confesses. "I've lost 30 pounds recently and still have 80 pounds to go, but this past week, I feel terrific and even sexy at 217 pounds. When I was 217 pounds a year ago, I felt like the ugliest, fattest, most disgusting person alive."

The Perils of Success

What few people tell you until you've started to lose weight is that success doesn't just have its joys: it also has its perils. Here are some of the biggest perils of success—some that can have you sprinting towards the closest Tim Horton's if you're not fully prepared to deal with them:

- **No longer having a goal to work toward.** "Reaching my goal was a really wonderful feeling, but it was definitely anti-climactic," admits Amy, who recently lost 67 pounds. "I remember thinking 'This is it?'" Kathryn recalls experiencing similar feelings after she lost 70 pounds: "I felt like something was missing because I wasn't working toward a goal anymore, it seemed. I had no more weight to lose. I spent over a year working my butt off to lose one or two pounds a week and now I'm just at a standstill. That was very hard for me at first."

- **Not knowing what to expect next.** "It felt great to reach my goal weight, but it was also a little scary," recalls Kathryn. "There was a feeling of 'what next' for a few weeks after I hit goal weight, but then I found my stride again when I formulated a new workout plan."

- **Fear of failure.** "Success scares the pants off me," admits Jill, who is halfway towards her goal of losing 120 pounds. "I have been down this road several times and something happens and my weight piles on again. I am petrified of this. People are really starting to notice my weight loss now, even asking me how much more weight I intend to lose, etc. I don't like it when that happens. It makes me feel very uncomfortable because I don't want to be seen as a failure in another year or two if the weight takes control again."

- **Not having a realistic body image yet.** Many women who lose significant amounts of weight find that it takes time for their body image to catch up with reality. (Some studies have shown

The Skinny

"It is a joy to be the size I am now, but there is also some peril involved. Sometimes I forget that I was once over-weight and then I will join in with my friends and eat junk food, thinking it's okay because I'm thin now. I can't have too many days like that if I want to maintain successfully. That's why I try to always keep in mind what it was like to be heavier. I've gained my weight back twice before and I could do it again if I don't watch myself."

— Kathryn, who recently lost 70 pounds

that it can take up to two years for a woman to gain a realistic idea of her body size and shape after she loses weight. Not surprisingly, these women tend to overestimate the size of their bodies.) Kathryn continues to struggle with body image concerns, despite the fact that she has maintained her weight loss for a number of months: "Sometimes I feel thin and sexy and pretty, but other times I get something I call 'phantom chin' where I feel like my double-chin is back, and I feel bloated and gross. Or I'll get paranoid and feel like I've gained some weight and start obsessing about it. Then I'll weigh myself and realize that nothing is different. It's really weird. It happens less and less, the longer I maintain my goal weight. So maybe this will eventually disappear altogether."

Mastering Maintenance

Kathryn doesn't pull any punches when she talks about what it takes to maintain a weight loss such as hers: "I think the real challenge is in keeping the weight off. A lot of us have become weight-loss masters over the years. We lose forty pounds one year, we gain it back. We lose thirty another year, then gain it back. I think we know what it takes to lose the weight or we wouldn't have been able to do it before. The real challenge is never gaining it back again. It's just like quitting smoking. It may be hard to quit, but how much harder is it never to smoke again?"

Amy agrees that weight maintenance comes with its own set of challenges, but she finds it easier than losing weight: "Maintaining can be difficult because you don't need to be quite so vigilant as you were during the weight-loss phase, and you don't have that constant reinforcement each week at the scales. However, if you can get into a pattern of eating that prevents you from feeling deprived, I think this part is easier. The reason most people find maintenance harder than losing is (in my opinion) because they never find the balance for themselves. They are constantly struggling to balance feelings of deprivation and the need to get what they want."

Here are some tips on mastering the art of maintaining your weight:

- **Don't deprive yourself.** "My number one secret is to never deprive myself," says Amy. "I always allow myself a little treat. I just make sure that I don't go overboard. I do this by monitoring my weight from week to week. If I have a gain for two consecutive weeks, I look back at my eating and figure out what I was doing in excess. Then I can correct the problem as it is happening. I found that after a few months of doing this, I don't seem to have a problem knowing how much I can treat myself without having to count calories or log a food diary."

- **Don't kid yourself.** Just as deprivation can spell disaster for anyone who's trying to maintain a weight loss, so can going overboard in the food department. It's important to remind yourself that you still have to watch your food intake, even if you're no longer trying to lose weight. Kathryn says, "It's hard to make people understand why I feel the need to be moderate when it comes to food. They don't understand that I'm pretty much battling an addiction, just as if I were a former smoker or a former alcoholic. It's tough."

- **Stay active.** It's hard to overstate the importance of remaining physically active after you've reached your goal weight. It's a lesson that Kathryn admits to having learned the hard way over the years: "I think what contributed to my weight-loss failures in the past was hating exercise. I looked at it as something I was forced to do in order to lose weight, but that I could quit doing once I lost the weight. I guess I thought, 'Wow, I'm thin. I don't have to worry about it anymore.' And that is simply not true. For me to be successful at weight maintenance, I need exercise in my life. I also see how much healthier exercise makes me. So this time around, I haven't stopped working out. I've gone out of my way to make exercise more enjoyable for me."

- **Pay attention to your body's early warning signals.** Don't wait until you've gained back 20 pounds before you start taking action. Be prepared to cut back your food intake and increase your exercise output as soon as the scale shows a five- to ten-pound gain. "It's all too easy for the pounds to creep back," notes Miriam

Food for Thought

Research has shown that people who have previously been obese have slower metabolisms than people who've never been obese. The difference? A hefty 15 percent.

Fat Chance

Think you can let that gym membership expire now that you've reached your goal? Think again. Studies have shown that you need more—not less—exercise after you lose weight. According to Thomas Wadden, Ph.D., director of the Weight and Eating Disorders Program at the University of Pennsylvania School of Medicine, your caloric needs drop by approximately 10 calories for every pound lost. You're therefore left with the choice of either cutting back the amount of food you eat or increasing the amount of exercise you get. Bottom line? You can figure on a minimum of three hours of heavy-duty aerobic exercise per week—and perhaps even more—if you're serious about keeping your weight down.

Nelson in *Strong Women Stay Slim*. "This can happen slowly. Since you might not notice a change in your clothing immediately, the scale provides the best early warning."

· **Have confidence in your ability to maintain your weight loss.** It's important to remind yourself that your weight-loss history won't necessarily repeat itself, notes Janis Jibrin in *The Unofficial Guide to Dieting Safely*. "Just because you've lost and gained a number of times before, it doesn't mean you will inevitably gain the weight back."

A Genuine Work in Progress

We may have come to the end of the book, but my weight-loss journey is far from over. (I'm well past the halfway point now, but I still can't quite see the 142 pound flag over the edge of the horizon!)

If you're just starting out on your own weight-loss journey and feeling like success is still miles away for you, remember that we're making this journey together. Each time you hit the gym on a day when you'd rather just flop out on the couch, or pour low-fat evaporated milk in your coffee when your body is shouting "cream," you can take heart in knowing that I'm probably doing the exact same thing. (Okay, I confess: Sometimes I can't resist the cream!)

If you'd like to drop me a line to tell me a bit about your own experiences as an Incredible Shrinking Woman, I'd love to hear from you. You can e-mail me at pageone@kawartha.com or write to me care of my publisher:

Ann Douglas
a.k.a. "The Incredible Shrinking Woman"
c/o Editorial Department – Professional, Trade and Reference Division
Prentice Hall Canada
26 Prince Andrew Place
Don Mills, Ontario M3C 2T8

P.S.: If you're disappointed that the book is finished—sometimes I feel that way when I come to the end of a book that I really liked—take heart:

The Skinny

"In the end, moving your body is not about flat stomachs or thin thighs; it's about being one of the three billion women on the planet who is lucky enough to have arms and legs that can surge with energy, be warmed by the sun, and slice through wind and water. Moving your body is about physically connecting with the fundamental joy and gratitude of being alive. The rest is gravy."

— Geneen Roth, *When You Eat at the Refrigerator, Pull Up a Chair*

you're not quite at the end yet! You'll find all kinds of neat stuff in the appendices that follow: a calorie and fat chart, a directory of weight-loss-related organizations, leads on the hottest places to tap into weight-loss advice online, a list of recommended readings, some delicious low-fat recipes, and a copy of a radio script I wrote for CBC Radio on what it's like to be a large woman in a world that worships thinness. (It's called "Larger Than Life" and you'll find it in Appendix D.)

Appendix A

Calorie Counts and Fat Gram Counts for Common Foods

While you don't want to become too obsessed with counting calories and fat grams, it can be useful to have a rough idea of how much food you're consuming over the course of a day. The following table includes calorie counts and fat gram counts for most common foods.

	CALORIES	FAT (GRAMS)
GRAIN PRODUCTS		
Bagel		
Plain (3")	163	1
Oat bran (3")	145	0.7
Biscuit (1 small)	105	5
Bread		
Crumbs (1 cup)	427	6
Italian (1 slice)	85	0
Mixed grain (1 slice)	80	1
Pita		
White (1, 6-1/2" diameter)	165	0.7
Whole wheat (1, 6-1/2" diameter)	170	1.7
Raisin (1 slice)	88	1.4
Rye (1 slice)	83	1
Sticks (1 small, 4-1/4" long)	21	0.5
White (1 slice)	75	1
Whole wheat (1 slice)	82	1
Pumpernickel (1 slice)	82	1
Cereal (also see Grains)		
Bran flakes (1 cup)	135	1
Cheerios (1 cup)	110	2
Corn Chex (1 cup)	111	0

	CALORIES	FAT (GRAMS)
Crispy rice (1 cup)	110	0
Farina, cooked (1 cup)	117	0
Grape Nuts (1/3 cup)	136	0
Granola, low-fat (1/3 cup)	110	2
Oat bran, cooked (1 cup)	88	2
Oatmeal, cooked (1 cup)	150	3
Oats, instant, cooked (1 cup)	138	2.3
Puffed rice, plain (1 cup)	50	0
Raisin Bran (1 cup)	174	1
Shredded Wheat (1 biscuit)	80	0
Total (1 cup)	100	1
Wheaties (1 cup)	101	1
Crackers		
Cheese, bite-size (1 cup)	312	16
Graham, low-fat (2)	110	2
Matzoh, plain (1)	112	0.4
Melba toast, plain, pieces (1 cup)	117	1
Rye, wafer, plain (1, 4-1/2" × 2-1/2")	37	0.1
Saltine, multi-grain (5)	60	2
Flour		
Buckwheat, whole groat (1 cup)	402	4
Cornmeal		
Degermed, white (1 cup)	505	2
Degermed, yellow (1 cup)	505	2
Whole-grain, white (1 cup)	441	4
Whole-grain, yellow (1 cup)	441	4
Cracker meal (1 cup)	440	2
Rice		
Brown (1 cup)	574	4
White (1 cup)	578	2
Rye		
Dark (1 cup)	415	3.5
Medium (1 cup)	361	2
Light (1 cup)	374	1.4
Wheat		
Durum (1 cup)	651	4.7
White (1 cup)	455	1.2
Whole-grain (1 cup)	407	2.2
Grains		
Barley, cooked (1 cup)	195	1

	CALORIES	FAT (GRAMS)
Buckwheat groats, roasted, cooked (1 cup)	155	1
Bulghur, cooked (1 cup)	150	0
Corn grits, cooked (1 cup)	145	0.5
Couscous, cooked (1 cup)	200	0
Hominy, canned (1 cup)	119	1.5
Millet, cooked (1 cup)	286	2.4
Rice		
Brown, cooked (1 cup)	216	2
White, cooked (1 cup)	264	1
Wild, cooked (1 cup)	166	0.6
Semolina, enriched (1 cup)	601	2
Wheat bran (2 tbsp.)	15	0
Wheat germ, toasted (2 tbsp.)	54	2
Whole wheat, cooked (1 cup)	150	1
Muffin		
Bran (1 small)	112	5
Corn (1 small)	125	4
English		
Plain (1)	134	1
Whole wheat (1)	134	1.4
Pancake (1 small)	60	2
Pasta		
Macaroni, cooked (1 cup)	183	1
Noodles, cooked (1 cup)	213	2
Noodles, egg (1 cup)	213	2.4
Spaghetti (1 cup)	182	0.9
Roll		
French (1)	105	2
Hard (1)	155	2
Snack		
Popcorn, plain, air-popped (1 cup)	25	0
Rice cake, regular (1)	35	0
Taco shell, baked (1, 6-1/2" diameter)	98	5
Tortillas		
Ready-to-bake, corn (6")	58	0.7
Ready-to-bake, flour (6")	104	2.3

	CALORIES	FAT (GRAMS)
VEGETABLES AND FRUIT		
Vegetables		
Artichokes (1 medium)	60	0.2
Asparagus, cooked (1/2 cup)	22	0
Beans, green, cooked (1/2 cup)	22	0
Beets, cooked, sliced (1/2 cup)	26	0
Broccoli, cooked (1/2 cup)	23	0
Brussels sprouts, cooked (1/2 cup)	30	0
Cabbage, raw, shredded (1 cup)	16	0
Carrot		
Grated (1 cup)	47	0.2
Whole (1 medium)	31	0
Cauliflower, cooked (1/2 cup)	15	0
Celery, raw (1 stalk)	6	0
Cucumber, slices (1/2 cup)	7	trace
Eggplant, cooked (1/2 cup)	23	0
Kale, cooked (1/2 cup)	21	0
Lettuce, raw, chopped (1 cup)	10	0
Mushrooms, sliced, cooked (1/2 cup)	21	0
Okra, cooked (1/2 cup)	34	0
Onion		
Yellow, cooked (1/2 cup)	30	0
Green, raw (1/2 cup)	13	0
Peas, green, cooked from frozen (1/2 cup)	63	0
Pepper, green, chopped, cooked (1/2 cup)	12	0
Potato		
White, baked, with skin (1 medium)	220	0
Sweet, baked, peeled (1 medium)	118	0
Radishes, raw (10)	7	0
Spinach		
Cooked (1/2 cup)	20	0
Raw (1 cup)	12	0
Squash		
Acorn, cooked, mashed (1/2 cup)	42	0
Zucchini, cooked (1/2 cup)	15	0
Sweet potato (1 medium)	158	0.5
Tomato		
Chopped (1/2 cup)	18	0
Whole (1)	24	0

	CALORIES	FAT (GRAMS)
Fruit		
Apple, medium (1)	81	1
Apple, dried, uncooked (1 cup)	209	0.3
Applesauce, unsweetened (1/2 cup)	53	0
Apple juice (1 cup)	116	0
Apricot (1)	17	0
Apricot, dried (1/4 cup)	77	0
Apricot nectar (1 cup)	141	0.2
Avocado, California (1)	306	30
Avocado, Florida (1)	341	27
Banana, medium (1)	105	1
Blackberries (1 cup)	75	0.6
Blueberries (1 cup)	81	1
Cherries, sweet (raw) (1 cup)	85	1
Cranberries (raw) (1 cup)	47	0.2
Cranberry juice cocktail (1 cup)	144	0
Cranberry sauce, sweetened (1/4 cup)	105	0
Currants		
European black, raw (1 cup)	71	0.5
Zante, dried (1 cup)	408	0.4
Dates, dry, chopped (1 cup)	490	0.8
Elderberries (1 cup)	106	0.7
Fig (1 medium, 2-1/4" diameter)	37	0.2
Fig, dried, uncooked (1)	49	0.2
Gooseberries, canned, light syrup (1 cup)	184	0.5
Grapefruit (1/2)	37	0
Grapefruit juice, unsweetened (1 cup)	94	0.3
Grapes		
American (slip skin) (1 cup)	58	0.3
European (adherent skin) (1 cup)	114	0.9
Grape juice, unsweetened (1 cup)	154	0.2
Guava (1 cup)	124	1.5
Kiwi (1)	45	0
Kumquats (1)	12	trace
Lemon juice (1 fl. oz.)	8	0
Lime juice (1 fl. oz.)	8	trace
Mango (1)	135	0.6
Melon		
Cantaloupe balls (1 cup)	62	0.5
Honeydew cubes (1 cup)	60	0

	CALORIES	FAT (GRAMS)
Nectarine (1)	67	1
Oranges		
California, Valencia (1, 2-5/8" diameter)	60	0.4
California, navel (1, 2-7/8" diameter)	64	0.1
Florida (1, 2-5/8" diameter)	65	0.3
Mandarin, canned in juice (1 cup)	92	0.1
Orange juice, fresh (1 cup)	112	1
Papaya, cut up (1 cup)	55	0
Papaya nectar (1 cup)	143	0.4
Passion-fruit (1)	18	0.1
Peach (1)	37	0
Peaches, dried, uncooked (1/2 cup)	31	0.1
Peach nectar (1 cup)	135	trace
Pears		
Bartlett (1)	98	1
Dried, uncooked (1/2 cup)	199	0.5
Persimmon (1)	32	0.1
Pineapple, cut up (1 cup)	76	1
Pineapple juice, unsweetened (1 cup)	140	0.2
Plantains, cooked, sliced (1 cup)	179	0.3
Plum (1)	36	0
Pomegranate (1, 3-3/8" diameter)	105	0.5
Prickly pear (1)	42	0.5
Prunes		
Dried, uncooked (1)	20	trace
Stewed (1/2 cup)	106	0
Prune juice (1 cup)	182	0.1
Quince (1)	52	0.1
Raisins (1/4 cup)	109	1
Raspberries (1 cup)	60	1
Rhubarb, cut up (1 cup)	26	0
Strawberries (1 cup)	45	1
Tangerine (1)	37	0
Watermelon, cut up (1 cup)	51	1

MILK PRODUCTS

Cheese

American (1 oz.)	106	9
Blue (1 oz.)	100	8

	CALORIES	FAT (GRAMS)
Brie (1 oz.)	95	8
Camembert (1 oz.)	85	7
Cheddar (1 oz.)	114	9
Colby (1 oz.)	112	9
Cottage		
1 percent low-fat (1 cup)	164	2
2 percent fat (1 cup)	203	4.4
Regular (1 cup)	234	10
Cream (1 tbsp.)	51	5
Edam (1 oz.)	101	8
Feta (1 oz.)	75	6
Goat cheese, semisoft (1 oz.)	103	8.5
Gouda (1 oz.)	101	8
Gruyere (1 oz.)	117	9.2
Limburger (1 oz.)	93	7.8
Monterey Jack (1 oz.)	106	9
Mozzarella		
Part skim milk (1 oz.)	72	4.6
Whole milk (1 oz.)	80	6.2
Muenster (1 oz.)	104	9
Neufchatel (1 oz.)	74	6.7
Parmesan, grated (1 oz.)	129	9
Port de salut (1 oz.)	100	8
Provolone (1 oz.)	100	8
Ricotta		
Part-skim (1/2 cup)	170	10
Whole milk (1/2 cup)	214	16
Romano (1 oz.)	110	8
Roquefort (1 oz.)	105	8.7
Swiss (1 oz.)	107	8
Ice Cream		
Chocolate (1/2 cup)	143	7.3
Strawberry (1/2 cup)	127	5.5
Vanilla		
Ice milk (1/2 cup)	92	2.9
Regular (1/2 cup)	133	7.3
Milk		
1 percent low-fat (1 cup)	102	3
2 percent (1 cup)	121	5
Buttermilk (1 cup)	99	2

	CALORIES	**FAT (GRAMS)**
Canned		
Condensed, sweetened (1 cup)	982	27
Evaporated, whole (1 fl. oz.)	43	2.4
Cream		
Half and half (1 tbsp.)	20	1.8
Sour		
Imitation (1 cup)	480	45
Regular, cultured (1 cup)	493	48
Regular, cultured (1 tbsp.)	26	2.5
Whipping		
Light, whipped (2 cups)	699	74
Heavy, whipped (2 cups)	821	88
Heavy (1 tbsp.)	37	3.8
Dry		
Skim (1 cup)	435	1
Whole (1 cup)	635	34
Goat (1 cup)	168	10
Skim (1 cup)	90	1
Whole (1 cup)	150	8
Yogurt		
Plain		
Nonfat (1 cup)	127	trace
Low-fat (1 cup)	144	4
Whole (1 cup)	139	7
MEAT AND ALTERNATIVES*		
Bacon, cooked (1 slice)	36	3
Beans		
Black, cooked (1/2 cup)	125	1
Fava, cooked (1 cup)	187	1
Garbanzo, cooked (1/2 cup)	143	1
Great northern, cooked (1 cup)	209	1
Kidney, cooked (1 cup)	225	1
Lima, cooked (1/2 cup)	94	0
Navy, cooked (1/2 cup)	129	1
Pinto, cooked (1/2 cup)	117	0
Soy, cooked (1 cup)	298	16
White, cooked (1 cup)	255	2

	CALORIES	**FAT (GRAMS)**
Beef		
Bottom round, cooked (3 oz.)	178	7
Flank steak, cooked (3 oz.)	176	9
Ground, lean (3 oz.)	230	15
Sirloin, cooked (3 oz.)	165	6
Top round, cooked (3 oz.)	153	4
Bologna (1 slice, 4" diameter × 1/8" thick)	71	6.6
Chicken		
White meat, cooked (3 oz.)	142	3
Drumstick, cooked (3 oz.)	151	5
Thigh, cooked (3 oz.)	163	7
Egg, whole (1 large)	75	5
Egg-white (1 large)	16	0
Egg-yolk (1 large)	59	5
Ham, cured, cooked (3 oz.)	140	6.5
Hot dog, beef (1)	142	13
Lamb		
Arm, cooked (3 oz.)	173	9
Leg, cooked (3 oz.)	162	7
Shank, cooked (3 oz.)	153	6
Lentils, cooked (1/2 cup)	115	0
Pork		
Centre loin, cooked (3 oz.)	204	11
Tenderloin, roasted, lean (3 oz.)	141	4
Seafood		
Catfish, cooked (3 oz.)	129	7
Clams, canned, drained (3 oz.)	126	2
Cod, cooked (3 oz.)	89	1
Crab, king, cooked (3 oz.)	82	1
Flounder, cooked (3 oz.)	99	1
Halibut, cooked (3 oz.)	119	3
Lobster, cooked (3 oz.)	84	1
Mackerel, cooked (3 oz.)	171	9
Monkfish, cooked (3 oz.)	82	2
Orange roughy, cooked (3 oz.)	75	1
Oysters, cooked (3 oz.)	116	4
Salmon		
Atlantic, cooked (3 oz.)	175	11
Coho, cooked (3 oz.)	151	7
Pink, canned (3 oz.)	114	5

	CALORIES	FAT (GRAMS)
Scallops, cooked (3 oz.)	75	1
Shrimp, cooked (3 oz.)	84	1
Snapper, cooked (3 oz.)	109	2
Surimi (imitation seafood) (3 oz.)	84	1
Swordfish, cooked (3 oz.)	132	4
Trout, rainbow, cooked (3 oz.)	128	5
Tuna		
Fresh, cooked (3 oz.)	156	5
White, canned in water (3 oz.)	90	1
Split peas, cooked (1/2 cup)	116	0
Tempeh (1 cup)	330	13
Tofu (3 oz.)	88	6
Turkey		
White meat, cooked (3 oz.)	115	1
Dark meat, cooked (3 oz.)	137	4
Veal		
Arm, cooked (3 oz.)	139	5
Rib, cooked (3 oz.)	150	6
Top round, cooked (3 oz.)	128	3

OTHER FOODS

Beverages: Alcohol

Beer		
Light (12 fl. oz.)	99	0
Regular (12 fl. oz.)	146	0
Distilled		
80-proof, gin, rum, vodka, whiskey (1 fl. oz.)	65	0
86-proof, gin, rum, vodka, whiskey (1 fl. oz.)	70	0
100-proof, all (1 fl. oz.)	82	0
Wine		
Red (3.5 fl. oz.)	74	0
Rosé (3.5 fl. oz.)	73	0
White (3.5 fl. oz.)	70	0

Beverages: Carbonated

Club soda (16 fl. oz.)	0	0
Cola		
Low-cal, w/aspartame (16 fl. oz.)	0	0
Regular (16 fl. oz.)	202	0
Ginger ale (16 fl. oz.)	166	0

	CALORIES	FAT (GRAMS)
Tonic water (16 fl. oz.)	114	0
Beverages: Coffee and Tea		
Coffee		
Brewed (8 fl. oz.)	4.8	0
Instant, decaffeinated (6 fl. oz.)	3.6	0
Instant, regular (6 fl. oz.)	3.6	0
Tea		
Brewed (8 fl. oz.)	2.4	0
Chamomile (8 fl. oz.)	2.4	0
Herb, other than chamomile (8 fl. oz.)	1.8	0
Condiments		
Ketchup (1 tbsp.)	16	trace
Pickles, dill (1 cup sliced)	28	0.3
Pickles, sweet (1 cup sliced)	199	0.4
Relish, green pickle (1 tbsp.)	20	trace
Fats and Oils		
Butter (1 tbsp.)	102	12
Chicken fat (1 tbsp.)	115	13
Lard (1 tbsp.)	115	13
Margarine (1 tbsp.)	102	11
Mayonnaise		
Low calorie (1 tbsp.)	40	4
Regular (1 tbsp.)	99	11
Oil		
Canola (1 tbsp.)	124	14
Corn (1 tbsp.)	120	14
Olive (1 tbsp.)	120	14
Peanut (1 tbsp.)	120	14
Sesame (1 tbsp.)	120	14
Soybean (1 tbsp.)	120	14
Salad dressing		
Blue cheese		
Low-calorie (1 tbsp.)	10	1
Regular (1 tbsp.)	77	8
French		
Low-calorie (1 tbsp.)	22	1
Regular (1 tbsp.)	67	6
Italian		
Low-calorie (1 tbsp.)	16	2
Regular (1 tbsp.)	69	7

	CALORIES	FAT (GRAMS)
Thousand Island		
Low-calorie (1 tbsp.)	24	2
Regular (1 tbsp.)	59	6
Vegetable oil cooking spray (1 spritz)	1–7	0–1
Nuts and Seeds		
Almonds, dry roasted (1 cup)	560	50
Brazil (1/4 cup)	230	29
Cashews, dry roasted (1/4 cup)	197	16
Macadamia, oil roasted (1/4 cup)	240	26
Peanuts, oil roasted (1/4 cup)	210	18
Peanut butter		
Chunky (2 tbsp.)	189	16
Smooth (1 tbsp.)	94	8
Pecans, dry roasted (1 oz.)	187	18
Pistachio, dry roasted (1/4 cup)	185	16
Pumpkin seeds, oil roasted (1/4 cup)	72	3
Sunflower seeds, oil roasted (1/4 cup)	208	20
Walnuts, chopped (1/4 cup)	190	18
Soy milk, fluid (1 cup)	81	5
Soy sauce (1 tbsp.)	11	trace

* Note: 4 ounces raw meat, poultry, or seafood generally yields 3 ounces cooked. Meat values are for lean portion only.

Sources: *The Complete Idiot's Guide to Losing Weight* by Susan McQuillan, M.S., R.D., with Edward Saltzman, M.D.; *The Dummies Guide to Dieting* by Jane Kirby, R.D.; *Eat More, Weigh Less* by Dean Ornish, M.D.

Appendix B
Directory of Fitness
and Weight-Loss-Related Organizations

CANADIAN ORGANIZATIONS

Bulimia Anorexia Nervosa Association
300 Cabana Rd. E
Windsor, ON N9G 1A3
Phone: (519) 969-2112
Fax: (519) 969-0227
Web: http://www.bana.ca
E-mail: info@bana.ca

Canadian Fitness and Lifestyle Research Institute
185 Somerset Street West, Suite 201
Ottawa, ON K2P 0J2
Phone: (613) 233-5528
Fax: (613) 233-5536
Web: http://www.cflri.ca
E-mail: info@cflri.ca

Canadian Institute of Stress
P.O. Box 665, Station "U"
Toronto, ON M8Z 5Y9
Phone: (416) 236-4218
Fax: (416) 237-9894
Web: http://www.stresscanada.org
E-mail: earle@idirect.com

Health Canada
A.L. 0913A
Ottawa, ON K1A 0K9
Phone: (613) 957-2991
Fax: (613) 941-5366
Web: http://www.hc-sc.gc.ca/english/
E-mail: info@www.hc-sc.gc.ca

Women's Health Office
Faculty of Health Sciences
Room 2B11
McMaster University
1200 Main Street West
Hamilton, ON L8N 3Z5
Phone: (905) 525-9140 ext. 22210
Fax: (905) 522-6898
Web: http://www-fhs.mcmaster.ca\women
E-mail: who@mcmaster.ca

National Eating Disorder Information Centre
CW 1-211, 200 Elizabeth Street
Toronto, ON M5G 2C4
Phone: (416) 340-4156
Fax: (416) 340-4736
Web: http://www.nedic.on.ca
E-mail: josullivan@torhosp.toronto.on.ca

National Institute of Nutrition
265 Carling Avenue, Suite 302
Ottawa, ON K1S 2E1
Phone: (613) 235-3355
Fax: (613) 235-7032
Web: http://www.nin.ca
E-mail: nin@nin.ca

YWCA Canada
590 Jarvis Street, 5th Floor
Toronto, ON M4Y 2J4
Phone: (416) 962-8881
Fax: (416) 962-8084
Web: http://www.ywcacanada.ca
E-mail: national@ywcacanada.ca

AMERICAN ORGANIZATIONS

American Anorexia/Bulimia Association Inc.
165 West 46th Street, Suite 1108
New York, NY 10036
Phone: (212) 575-6200
Fax: (212) 278-0698
Web: http://www.aabainc.org
E-mail: info@aabainc.org

American College of Sports Medicine
P.O. Box 1440
Indianapolis, IN 46206-1440
Phone: (317) 637-9200
Fax: (317) 634-7817
Web: http://www.acsm.org
E-mail: pipacsm@acsm.org

American Dietetic Association
216 West Jackson Boulevard
Chicago, IL 60606-6995
Phone: (900) 225-5267 (Nutrition Hotline)
       (800) 877-1600 ext. 5000 (Publications)
       (312) 899-0040
Fax: (312) 899-4899
Web: http://www.eatright.org
E-mail: webmaster@eatright.org

American Obesity Association
1250 24th Street, NW
Suite 300
Washington, DC 20037
Phone: 800-98-OBESE (986-2373)
       (202) 776-7711 (in DC)
Fax: (202) 776-7712
Web: http://www.obesity.org

American Running and Fitness Association
4405 East-West Highway
Suite 405
Bethesda, MD 20814-4535
Phone: 800-776-ARFA (2732)
       (301) 913-9517
Fax: (301) 913-9520
Web: http://www.arfa.org
E-mail: arfaun@aol.com

American Society for Bariatric Surgery
140 NW 75th Drive
Suite C
Gainesville, FL 32607
Phone: (352) 331-4900
Fax: (352) 331-4975
Web: http://www.asbs.org
E-mail: Mallorygn@asbs.org

American Society of Bariatric Physicians
5600 South Quebec Street
Suite 109-A
Englewood, CO 80111
Phone: (303) 779-4833 (automated referral line)
       (303) 770-2526
Fax: (202) 779-4834
Web: http://www.asbp.org
E-mail: bariatric@asbp.org

Council on Size and Weight Discrimination Inc.
P.O. Box 305
Mount Marion, NY 12456
Phone: (914) 679-1209
Fax: (914) 679-1206
E-mail: councilswd@aol.com

Eating Disorders Awareness and Prevention Inc.
603 Stewart Street, Suite 803
Seattle, WA 98101
Phone: (800) 931-2237
       (206) 382-3587 (in WA)
Fax: 206-292-9890

Food and Drug Administration
Office of Consumer Affairs
5600 Fishers Lane
Rockville, MD 20857
Phone: 888-INFO-FDA (463-6332)
Fax: 301-443-9767
Web: http://www.fda.gov
E-mail: webmail@oc.fda.gov

Food and Nutrition Information Center
USDA, National Agricultural Library
10301 Baltimore Avenue, Room 304
Beltsville, MD 20705-2351
Phone: (301) 504-5719
Fax: (301) 504-6409
TTY: (301) 504-6856 (TTY)
Web: http://www.nal.usda.gov/fnic
E-mail: fnic@nal.usda.gov

International Food Information Council Foundation
1100 Connecticut Avenue, NW, Suite 430
Washington, DC 20036
Phone: (202) 296-6540
Fax: (202) 296-6547
Web: http://ificinfo.health.org
E-mail: foodinfo@ific.health.org

National Association of Anorexia Nervosa and
Associated Disorders
P.O. Box 7
Highland Park, IL 60035
Phone: (847) 831-3438
Fax: (847) 433-4632
E-mail: anad20@aol.com

National Association to Advance Fat Acceptance
P.O. Box 188620
Sacramento, CA 95818
Phone: (916) 558-6880
Fax: (916) 558-6881
Web: http://naafa.org
E-mail: naafa@naafa.org

National Center for Health Statistics
Data Dissemination Branch
6525 Belcrest Rd., Room 1064
Hyattsville, MD 20782
Phone: (301) 436-8500
Web: http://www.cdc.gov/nchswww
E-mail: nchsquery@cdc.gov

National Health Information Center
P.O. Box 1133
Washington, DC 20013-1133
Phone: (800) 336-4797
    (301) 565-4167
Fax: (301) 984-4256
Web: http://nhic-nt.health.org
E-mail: nhicinfo@health.org

Shape Up America
6707 Democracy Blvd.
Suite 306
Bethesda, MD 20817
Phone: (301) 493-5368
Fax: (301) 493-9504
Web: http://www.shapeup.org
E-mail: suainfo@shapeup.org

U.S. Department of Agriculture
Cooperative State Research, Education, and Extension
Service
14th and Independence Avenue, SW
Rm. 304A, Whitten Bldg.
Washington, DC 20250
Phone: (202) 720-4423
Fax: (202) 720-8987
Web: http://www.usda.gov
E-mail: webmaster@fns.usda.gov

Weight-Control Information Network
1 Win Way
Bethesda, MD 20892-3665
Phone: (301) 984-7378
Fax: (301) 984-7196
Web: http://www.niddk.nih.gov/health/nutrit/win.htm
E-mail: win@info.niddk.nih.gov

Appendix C
Web Site Directory

If you have access to the Internet, your weight-loss journey just got a whole lot easier. Here are some sites you'll definitely want to check out.

WEB SITE	HIGHLIGHTS
Fitness Information	
Canadian Fitness and Lifestyle Research Institute	
http://www.cflri.ca/cflri/cflri.html	This site is packed with valuable information about the fitness habits of Canadians.
Health Canada	
http://www.paguide.com	You can download your own copy of *Canada's Guide to Physical Activity* and pick up other valuable fitness-related information by visiting this site.
Phys.com	
http://www.phys.com	A terrific source of fitness and weight-loss-related information. Definitely worth a visit.
Health Information	
C-Health	
http://www.canoe.ca/Health/home.html	The health section of the huge and growing Canadian News Online (CANOE) Web site. Features news, columns, and more.
Healthy Way	
http://www1.sympatico.ca/healthyway/	Canada's largest health-related Web site. Contains links to all kinds of useful information on a variety of health-related topics, including fitness and nutrition.
Mayo Health Oasis (Mayo Clinic)	
http://www.mayohealth.org	Features meticulously researched articles on a smorgasbord of health-related topics, including fitness and nutrition.
Mediconsult	
http://www.mediconsult.com	Another one of the big U.S. health Web sites. Features a variety of online support groups, the latest medical news, and a whole lot more.
Medline	
http://www.nlm.nih.gov/ databases/freemedl.html	A database that allows you to search for abstracts from the latest medical journals. An essential tool for the slightly obsessed weight watcher who wants to know everything possible about fitness and nutrition!

WEB SITE	HIGHLIGHTS
WebMD http://www.webmd.com	One of the best health Web sites out there. Contains the latest news on both diet and nutrition and sports and fitness.
Nutrition Information	
Tufts University Nutrition Navigator http://www.navigator.tufts.edu	Provides links to the best nutrition-related Web sites online. You can find their picks of the best sites for women at http://www.navigator.tufts.edu/women.html
Weight-Loss Information	
National Weight Loss Control Registry http://www.uchsc.edu/ nutrition/nwcr.htm	Find out about the National Weight Loss Control Registry, a database of people who have successfully maintained weight losses of 60 pounds or more for at least five years.
Prevention http://www.prevention.com/weight/	The official Web site for *Prevention* magazine. Contains plenty of useful articles on fitness and weight loss.
Weight-Loss Support	
CyberDiet http://www.cyberdiet.com	The Cadillac of weight-loss support sites, CyberDiet offers everything from message boards to weight-loss tools to access to online chats.
Diet Riot http://www.dietriot.com	Contains an interesting mix of weight-loss-related information and fun stuff, like diet greeting cards!
The Incredible Shrinking Woman http://www.sanitysavers.com/incredible	The official Web site for this book. Drop by and introduce yourself!
IVillage Diet and Fitness http://www.ivillage.com/fitness/	Among the features of this information-packed Web site is the "Never Say Diet" weight-loss area. Definitely worth checking out.
Onelist.com http://www.onelist.com	Home to thousands of mailing lists. You can either find a weight-loss support group mailing list to join or you can start your own.
Three Fat Chicks http://www.3fatchicks.com	This site is the brainchild of three sisters (the so-called "fat chicks") who are trying to lose weight. It dishes up a unique blend of information and support.

Note: Don't forget to check out the many excellent Web sites that are listed in Appendix B. Some are them are nothing short of online encyclopedias!

Appendix D

Larger Than Life*

by Ann Douglas

Scene 1: Gym

1. SOUND:	*SOUNDS OF A GYM: AEROBIC INSTRUCTOR CALLING OUT INSTRUCTIONS. MUSIC WITH THROBBING BEAT. FADES TO SOUNDS OF SOMEONE RUNNING ON A TREAD-MILL OR USING AN EXERCISE BIKE.*
OLDER NARRATOR:	I never thought I'd live to see the day when I'd agree to join a gym—to fork over my hard-earned cash so I could take my plus-sized body out and sweat in public. But that's exactly what has happened. I, Ann Douglas, woman of size, recently joined a gym. And for the first time in my life, I am exercising not to lose weight, but rather because I want to feel strong and healthy.
	At first I worried that the place would be dominated by a bunch of Jane Fonda-clones in clingy leotards. Fortunately, that has not turned out to be the case. For every Kate Moss lookalike, there are a good dozen or so of us voluptuous, full-figured gals.
2. SOUND:	*ELECTRONIC BEEPS AS THREE DIGITS ARE KEYED INTO STAIRMASTER EQUIPMENT.*
OLDER NARRATOR:	I key my weight into the high-tech exercise machines. So what if the Stairmaster likes to flash my weight to the world in four-inch high neon letters—a futile attempt by some exercise-Nazi in the Stairmaster factory to keep us plus-sized gals in our place. I'm not intimidated!
3. SOUND:	*SOUND OF SOMEONE STEPPING ON AND OFF A SCALE.*
OLDER NARRATOR:	My weight is just a number. It's taken me years to get to the point where I can say that—to honestly believe that my weight has no more bearing on my worthiness as a person than my shoe size, my height, or the colour of my hair. In fact, it's taken me my entire life—35 years—to put the scale in its place and to stop wearing my weight like a scarlet letter.

*A version of this radio play was broadcast on October 29, 1999, on CBC Radio's *Outfront*.

Scene 2: Delivery Room in a Hospital

4. SOUND/MUSIC: *SOUND OF A DOCTOR ANNOUNCING, "IT'S A GIRL." THEN THE SOUND OF A NEWBORN BABY CRYING. FADE TO A LULLABY.*

OLDER NARRATOR: I had my first encounter with a scale a little over 35 years ago. I weighed in at a mere 5 lbs. 13 oz.—the one and only time in my life I would ever be classified as underweight.

By the time I got home from the hospital, I was well on my way to catching up with my heftier peers.

The cute chubby thighs that relatives found so engaging during my first few years had become a bit passé by the time I started school. It was a crime to be a fat kid.

Scene 3: Younger Narrator's Bedroom

5. SOUND/MUSIC: *"ALL BY MYSELF" BY ERIC CARMEN.*

YOUNGER NARRATOR: June 1973. It is track and field day at school today, but I get to stay home because of my eye operation. Not wanting to die because nobody will pick me for their team—or waiting for the laughs when I land on the bar during high jump. I get to miss high jump, long jump, shot put, and the relay race. I get to miss it all!

OLDER NARRATOR: I get to miss it all!

YOUNGER NARRATOR: Easter Sunday, 1974—The Easter Bunny came last night and brought something for each of the kids in the family. Janet, Lorna, and Sandra got big chocolate bunnies. I got a skipping rope.

OLDER NARRATOR: Just what I wanted.

6. SOUND/MUSIC: *"ALL BY MYSELF."*

YOUNGER NARRATOR: Fall 1975. Mom ordered me some new clothes from the Sears catalogue. They're supposed to be jeans, but they're made out of this shiny stretchy fabric and they have an elastic waist. They don't make normal jeans in the chubby sizes. I must be the only kid who's too big to wear regular jeans.

Of course, it's all my fault. I've got to stop eating chocolate chip cookies every time I'm alone in the kitchen. I've got to stop buying candy at the variety store. I've got to lose weight so I can wear normal clothes, so I can be a normal kid.

OLDER NARRATOR: That's all I ever wanted to be: a normal kid.

Scene 4: Shopping Mall

7. SOUND: *MALL MUSIC AND SOUNDS OF CASH REGISTERS.*

OLDER NARRATOR: We've come a long way when it comes to plus-sized clothing, baby, but not quite far enough. I live in a city of 70 000, and there's only one plus-sized clothing store for women. To make matters worse, there's nowhere to buy decent quality undergarments. The last time I made the trek to Ottawa to shop in a plus-sized lingerie store, I mentioned to the clerk that I'd travelled three hours to buy underwear and bras. She asked what the other women in my city did for underwear. I whispered slyly, "We've learned to do without."

Scene 5: Younger Narrator's Bedroom

8. SOUND/MUSIC: *"ALL BY MYSELF."*

YOUNGER NARRATOR: Summer 1976. I'm going to lose weight this summer so all the boys will think I'm as pretty as LeeAnn and Nancy. I'm going to swim from our dock to the Bakers' dock 50 times each day. I won't eat anything sugary, no matter how hungry I feel. It will be hard, but it will all be worth it.

A bunch of us drove out to Milton in Pete's father's car today. We stopped for a snack at McDonald's on the way. Everyone else had burgers and fries, but I just had a cup of coffee. I was hungry, but there was no way I was going to eat anything fattening in front of everyone else. What would they think if they saw me eating regular food?

Scene 6: TV Talk Show Set

9. SOUND: *SOUNDS OF TV CREW GETTING READY TO GO ON AIR. DOING SOUND CHECKS, ETC. THEN FADE TO SONG, "I DON'T WANT HER, YOU CAN HAVE HER, SHE'S TOO FAT FOR ME."*

OLDER NARRATOR: From time to time, I still get hit with an overwhelming urge to lose a ton of weight overnight. It usually happens when I've got to do a TV appearance to flog one of my books. The moment I start fixating on how I'm going to look in front of the camera, I get this overwhelming urge to starve myself, run around the block, and basically do whatever it takes to burn off fat in a hurry.

Then, after freaking out for a few moments, I get real. I remind myself that there are lots of large women on the talk show circuit. Heck, two of the most famous talk show hosts on TV today are plus-sized. (Take a bow Oprah and Rosie!) Either the world is finally becoming a safe place for women of size, or folks at two of the big U.S. networks have been asleep at the switch.

Scene 7: Younger Narrator's Bedroom

10. SOUND/MUSIC: *"ALL BY MYSELF."*

YOUNGER NARRATOR: Winter 1977. My family doctor just put me on a diet so I can lose about 30 pounds. It's only 800 calories per day, which means that I'm hungry a lot. In fact, I can't think of anything else but food. Sometimes I wake up in the middle of the night after dreaming about chocolate chip cookies and ice cream and bread with lots and lots of butter on it. At first I feel guilty for eating, but then I realize that I only ate them in my dreams. There are no calories in dreams.

I spend a lot of time thinking about calories—wondering what would happen if I ate a medium-sized apple rather than a small one and trying to decide if an orange has more than 40 calories if you're hungry enough to eat the peel.

When I'm really hungry, I chew gum. I chew it so much that my teeth get sore. Sometimes I wonder if you can actually get more than 4.7 calories out of a stick of sugarfree gum if you work at it long enough. You know what? Some kids in my class don't even know what a calorie is.

Scene 8: Monologue of Older Narrator

11. SOUND: *CLIPS FROM VARIOUS DIET COMMERCIALS: WEIGHT WATCHERS, JENNY CRAIG, ETC. FADE TO SOUND OF SOMEONE STEPPING ON AND OFF A SCALE.*

OLDER NARRATOR: I don't diet anymore. I've learned over the years that dieting doesn't work. Sure, the pounds come off initially, but when I get tired of eating a hard boiled egg for breakfast, tuna and melba toast for lunch, and a boiled chicken breast for dinner, the pounds come back with a vengeance.

That's not to say that I haven't tried my fair share of diets over the years. Heck, I've probably tried them all. And I've put enough money into Weight Watchers' coffers over the years to keep my chequing account suitably lean.

12. MUSIC: *"MISS AMERICA" THEME.*

OLDER NARRATOR: In July of 1987, the impossible happened: I reached my goal weight. But then I got pregnant the next month and gained back all the weight I had lost.

13. SOUND: *DOCTOR'S VOICE ANNOUNCES, "IT'S A GIRL." NEWBORN CRY. "IT'S A BOY." NEWBORN CRY. "IT'S A BOY." NEWBORN CRY. "IT'S ANOTHER BOY." NEWBORN CRY.*

OLDER NARRATOR: There were three more babies—and a lot more pounds—over the next ten years. After my first child was born, I just couldn't get all that enthused about weighing vegetables on a food scale anymore. When forced to choose between snatching an hour of sleep on the couch while my baby dozed in the baby swing or weighing a piece of broccoli, I succumbed to the magnetic pull of the couch.

14. MUSIC: *HELEN REDDY'S "I AM WOMAN."*

OLDER NARRATOR: Ironically, it was then that I started to give my body some grudging respect, extra pounds and all.

YOUNGER NARRATOR: You mean you started to like your body?

OLDER NARRATOR: The whole process started when I was pregnant. I loved knowing that there was a baby growing in me—feeling my baby's flutters and kicks and laying in the tub watching as the baby shifted from one side of my body to the other. *My* baby cradled in *my* body. For the first time in my life, I called a truce with my body—forgave it for being the size and shape it was. How could I hate my body when it was busy performing a miracle?

There are, of course, fringe benefits to being pregnant. You're supposed to have a huge belly. It just goes with the turf! What's more, everyone thinks you're cute and adorable. Your huge belly makes your thunder thighs look positively svelte. Of course, pregnancy is only a temporary solution—unless, of course, you plan to have one heck of a large family.

Scene 9: Schoolyard

15. SOUND: *GROUP OF CHILDREN TAUNTING: "FATTY, FATTY, TWO BY FOUR, COULDN'T GET THROUGH THE BATHROOM DOOR, SO SHE DID IT ON THE FLOOR. FATTY, FATTY, TWO BY FOUR." FADE TO SOUNDS OF CHILDREN LAUGHING AND PLAYING.*

OLDER NARRATOR: The more things change the more they stay the same. My nine-year-old came from school today and announced that one of the kids in her class says that I'm too fat. Actually, the kid didn't quite put in that politely. She said that I'm so fat that I take over the entire world.

My first reaction was to feel sick inside. My next reaction was to pick up the phone and call the kid's mother.

16. SOUND: *PHONE DIALING.*

OLDER NARRATOR: There are still a lot of battles to be won on the plus-sized front and I'm quite prepared to fight them. Just call me the plus-sized vigilante—a non-content who lets clothing manufacturers know that it's not okay that every large woman in town has to wear the same style of dress because there's only one place to shop for plus-sized clothing; who insists that airlines either make the economy class airline seats a little wider or let large people ride in the executive class for the same price; and who lets everyone know in no uncertain terms that open season on fat people is over, once and for all.

17. SOUND:	*PHONE RINGING. THEN FEMALE VOICE SAYS, "HELLO."*

OLDER NARRATOR:

I get lucky. The mother is a nice person, someone who is genuinely horrified to hear what her daughter had to say. She speaks to her daughter and the insults stop.

Today, Peterborough. Tomorrow, the world....

End.

Appendix E
Bibliography

Books

Angier, Natalie. *Woman: An Intimate Geography*. New York: Houghton Mifflin, 1999.

Bailey, Covert. *The Fit or Fat Woman: Solutions for Women's Unique Concerns*. Boston: Houghlin Mifflin, 1989.

Douglas, Ann. *Sanity Savers: The Canadian Working Woman's Guide to Almost Having It All*. Toronto: McGraw-Hill Ryerson Ltd., 1999.

Estrich, Susan.*Making the Case for Yourself: A Diet Book for Smart Women*. New York: Riverhead Books, 1997.

Etcoff, Nancy. *Survival of the Prettiest: The Science of Beauty*. New York: Doubleday, 1999.

Fletcher, Anne M. *Eating Thin for Life: Food Secrets and Recipes from People Who Have Lost Weight and Kept It Off*. New York: Houghton Mifflin, 1997.

Fletcher, Anne M. *Thin for Life: 10 Keys to Success from People Who Have Lost Weight and Kept It Off*. Shelburne, Vermont: Chapters Publishing, 1994.

Fraser, Laura. *Losing It: False Hopes and Fat Profits in the Diet Industry*. New York: Penguin Books, 1997.

Gullo, Stephen P. *Thin Tastes Better: Control Your Food Triggers Without Feeling Deprived*. New York: Dell Publishing, 1995.

Heber, David. *The Resolution Diet*. New York: Avery Publishing Group, 1999.

Hope, Jackqueline. *Big, Bold and Beautiful: Living Large on a Small Planet*. Toronto: Macmillan Canada, 1996.

Irons, Diane. *The World's Best-Kept Diet Secrets*. Napierville, IL: Sourcebooks, Inc., 1998.

Jibrin, Janis. *The Unofficial Guide to Dieting Safely*. Chicago, IL: IDG Books, 1998.

Kirby, Jane, R.D. *Dieting for Dummies*. Chicago, IL: IDG Books, 1998.

Lindsay, Anne. *Lighthearted Everyday Cooking*. Toronto: Macmillan Canada, 1991.

Lindsay, Anne. *The Lighthearted Cookbook*. Toronto: Macmillan Canada, 1988.

Lutter, Judy Mahle and Lynn Jaffee. *The Bodywise Woman*. Champaign, IL: Human Kinetics, 1996.

Manheim, Camryn. *Wake Up, I'm Fat*. New York: Broadway Books, 1999.

Marx, Patricia, and Susan Sistrom. *The Skinny: What Every Skinny Woman Knows About Dieting (And Won't Tell You!)*. New York: Dell Publishing, 1999.

McQuillan, Susan, M.S., R.D. with Edward Saltzman, M.D. *The Complete Idiot's Guide to Losing Weight*. New York: Alpha Books, 1998.

Mellin, Laurel. *The Solution*. New York: Harper Collins, 1997.

Nelson, Miriam, with Sarah Wernick, Ph.D. *Strong Women Stay Slim*. New York: Bantam Books, 1999.

Neporent, Liz, and Suzanne Schlosberg. *Weight Training for Dummies*. Chicago, IL: IDG Books, 1997.

Omichinski, Linda, and Heather Wiebe Hildebrand. *Tailoring Your Tastes*. Winnipeg: Tamos Books Inc., 1995.

Omichinski, Linda. *You Count, Calories Don't*. Winnipeg: Hyperion Press, 1992.

Ornish, Dean. *Eat More, Weigh Less*. New York: HarperCollins, 1993.

Oswald, Christopher A. *Stretching for Fitness, Health, and Performance*. New York: Sterling Publishing Co., 1998.

Podleski, Janet and Greta. *Crazy Plates*. Waterloo, Ontario: Granet Publishing Inc., 1999.

____. *Looneyspoons*. Waterloo, Ontario: Granet Publishing Inc., 1997.

Poulton, Terry. *No Fat Chicks: How Women Are Brainwashed to Hate Their Bodies and Spend Their Money*. Toronto: Key Porter Books, 1996.

Roth, Geneen. *Breaking Free from Compulsive Eating*. New York: Penguin Books USA, 1984.

____. *Feeding the Hungry Heart*. New York: Penguin Books USA, 1982.

____. *When Food Is Love*. New York: Penguin Books USA, 1989.

____. *When You Eat at the Refrigerator, Pull Up a Chair*. New York: Hyperion, 1999.

____. *Why Weight? A Guide to Ending Compulsive Eating*. New York: Penguin Books USA, 1989.

Schlosberg, Suzanne, and Liz Neporent. *Fitness for Dummies*. Chicago, IL: IDG Books, 1996.

Stearns, Peter N. *Fat History. Bodies and Beauty in the Modern West*. New York: New York University Press, 1997.

Articles and Pamphlets

"Being overweight can shorten your life, study says." CNN.com, October 6, 1999: Health.

"Body News." *Prevention's Guide—Weight Loss*, October 1999: 4.

"Body News." *Prevention's Guide—Weight Loss*, October 1999: 8.

"Dieters need intensive support during holidays." *Health Psychology*, July 9, 1999.

"Drink More, Breathe Easier." *Prevention*, November 1999: 70.

"Exercise: A Wise Investment for Women with PMS." *PMS Access*, Women's Health America Group, Madison, WI.

Barr, Richard B., EdD. "Exercising to Lose 10 to 20 Pounds." *The Physician and Sportsmedicine*, Vol. 25, No. 4, April 1997.

Barr, Richard B., EdD. "Exercising When You're Overweight: Getting in Shape and Shedding Pounds." *The Physician and Sportsmedicine*, Vol. 24, No. 10, October 1996.

Barrett, Cindy. "The Macho Workout Women Love." *Canadian Living*, September 1999: 69–72.

Bates, Colleen Dunn. "Seven Strategies for Permanent Change." *Shape*, October 1999: 24.

Brink, P.J., and K. Ferguson. "The decision to lose weight." *West J Nurs Res*, February 1998; 20(1): 84–102.

Burcum, Jill. "Diet Right? The surfeit of best-selling diet books is hard to ignore, but nutrition experts caution that some diets may not live up to their claims and could be harmful." *Minneapolis Star Tribune*, April 21, 1999: 01E.

Canada's Food Guide to Healthy Eating. Ottawa: Government of Canada, 1992.

Canada's Physical Activity Guide. Ottawa: Government of Canada, 1998.

Connell, Laura. "Easing The Agony of PMS." *Homemaker's*, October 1999: 148.

Craig, Cora Lynn, Storm J. Russell, Christine Cameron, and Angele Beaulieu. *Foundation for Joint Action. Reducing Physical Inactivity*. Ottawa: Canadian Fitness and Lifestyle Institute, 1999.

Curran, Victoria. "Winter Workout Boosters." *Canadian Living*, November 1999: 75–80.

Dann, Moira. "French Fries, Canada's favourite food." *The Globe and Mail*, June 30, 1999, A22.

David, Cynthia. "New Year, New You: 40 Diet Tips That Really Work." *Canadian Living*, Holiday 1999: 43, 45, 47–48.

Dye, L., and J.E. Blundell. "Menstrual cycle and appetite control: implications for weight regulation." *Human Reproduction*, June 1997; 12(6): 1142–51.

Federal Trade Commission. "Facts for Consumers: The Skinny on Dieting." http://www.ftc.gov/bcp/conline/pubs/health/diets.htm, March 1997.

Federal Trade Commission. "Setting Goals for Weight Loss." http://www.ftc.gov/bcp/conline/pubs/health/setgoals.htm, February 1999.

Fields, Julie. "Warnings to a fat nation." *The Record Online*, October 27, 1999, www.bergen.com:80.

"Food fantasies can be fattening." *Peterborough Examiner*, September 22, 1999, C1.

French, S.A., and R.W. Jeffery. "Current dieting, weight loss history, and weight suppression: behavioral correlates of three dimensions of dieting." *Addiction Behavior*, January/February 1997; 22(1): 31–44.

Fumento, Michael. "Living off the fat of the land: the only people benefiting from diet books are the authors." *Washington Monthly*, November 1, 1998: 40(3).

Ganske, Mary Garner. "5 myths that keep you from losing." *Redbook*, Vol. 190, March 1, 1998: 48(2).

Golin, Mark. "30 pounds down ... now and forever! How to make slimming lifestyle changes that really last a lifetime." *Prevention*, Vol. 46, January 1, 1994: 42(13).

Gotthardt, Melissa. "50 Ways to Survive the Fat Season." *Prevention*, November 1999: 138–145.

Grunwald, Lisa. "Discovery: Do I Look Fat to You? 28 Questions (and all the Answers) about our national obsession." *Life*, February 1, 1995: 58+.

Hammock, Delia A. "Trick Picks: Diet Foods That Can Wreck Your Diet." *Good Housekeeping*, October 1999: 147–148.

Hart, Diane. "The Busy Woman Workout." *Canadian Living*, June 1999: 125–127.

Health Canada. "Canadians and Health Eating: how are we doing?" *Nutrition Highlights, National Population Health Survey*, 1994–95, March 1997.

Health Letter Associates, University of California at Berkeley Wellness Letter. "Calculating your caloric needs." *The Globe and Mail*, July 13, 1999, C7.

Healthlines. "Ladies, Start Your Vacuums." *Homemaker's*, October 1999: 142.

Heinzl, John. "Marketers go one supersize up." *Report on Business*, June 30, 1999, M1.

Hirshorn, Susan. "Study Finds Link Between Stress and Fat." *Canadian Living*, October 1999: 21.

"How to assess weight-loss programs." *Consumers' Research Magazine*, January 1, 1995: 18(6).

International Food Information Council Foundation. *Food Insight*, July/August 1999.

Keeler, Helen. "Shins in Shape." *Canadian Living*, July 1999: 81.

Keller, Colleen, Deborah Oveland, and Staria Hudson. "Strategies for weight control success in adults." *The Nurse Practitioner*, Vol. 22, March 1, 1997: 33(8).

Keough, Kathleen. "Weight loss: Find the weight that's right for you." *Heart & Soul*, July 31, 1995: PG.

Kesterton, Michael. "Calcium and weight loss." *The Globe and Mail*, July 14, 1999, A16.

Kesterton, Michael. "How much exercise?" *The Globe and Mail*, November 17, 1999, A24.

Klem, M.L. et al. "A descriptive study of individuals successful at long-term maintenance of substantial weight loss." *American Journal of Clinical Nutrition*, August 1997; 66(2): 239–46.

Kurzer, M.S. "Women, food, and mood." *Nutrition Review*, July 1997; 55(7): 268–76.

Larkin, Marilyn. "Behavior, not biology, is key to weight loss." http://www.adam.com/news/462523.html, August 11, 1999.

Larkin, Marilyn. "Losing Weight Safely." *FDA Consumer*, Vol. 30, January 1, 1996.

Linton, Marilyn. "Extreme Dieting/From Cabbage Soup to Eggs All Day, Fad Diets Are Boring and Unhealthy." *The Toronto Sun*, August 29, 1999: 52.

Lowe, Eric Benjamin. "Blocking the binge: UF researchers explore treatment for uncontrolled eating." *University of Florida Health Newsnet*, August 8, 1999.

Lowe, Eric Benjamin. "UF researchers explore gene therapy to treat obesity." *University of Florida Health Newsnet*, June 10, 1999.

"Modest Weight Loss Helps." *Peterborough Examiner*, December 8, 1999: C3.

Nelson, Miriam E., Ph.D. "Does when you work out determine how many calories you burn?" CNN.com, July 14, 1999: Health.

Nelson, Miriam E., Ph.D. "Eating before exercise: The facts." CNN.com, June 11, 1999: Health.

Nichols, Mark with Shaune MacKinlay. "The Obesity Epidemic: About half of all adult Canadians are overweight or obese—and the bill for treating the resulting diseases comes to an estimated $15 billion a year." *Maclean's*, January 11, 1999: 54.

NIDDK Weight-Control Information Network. *Choosing a Safe and Successful Weight-Loss Program*. NIH Publication, December 1993: 94-3700.

NIDDK Weight-Control Information Network. *Dieting and Gallstones*. NIH Publication, November 1993: 94-3677.

NIDDK Weight-Control Information Network. *Do You Know the Health Risks of Being Overweight?* NIH Publication, May 1998: 98-4098.

NIDDK Weight-Control Information Network. *Gastric Surgery for Severe Obesity*. NIH Publication, April 1996: 96-4006.

NIDDK Weight-Control Information Network. *Physical Activity and Weight Control*. NIH Publication, April 1996: 96-4031.

NIDDK Weight-Control Information Network. *Prescription Medications for the Treatment of Obesity*. NIH Publication, December 1996: 97-4191.

NIDDK Weight-Control Information Network. *Understanding Adult Obesity*. NIH Publication, November 1993: 94-3680.

NIDDK Weight-Control Information Network. *Very Low-Calorie Diets*. NIH Publication, March 1995: 95-3894.

NIDDK Weight-Control Information Network. *Walking...A Step in the Right Direction*. NIH Publication, October 1996: 97-4155.

NIDDK Weight-Control Information Network. *Weight Cycling*. NIH Publication, March 1995:95-3901.

NIDDK Weight-Control Information Network. *Do You Know the Health Risks of Being Overweight?* The National Institute of Diabetes and Digestive and Kidney Diseases, October 18, 1999.

Ohlin, A. and S. Rossner. "Factors related to body weight changes during and after pregnancy: the Stockholm Pregnancy and Weight Development Study." *Obes Res*, May 1996; 4(3): 271–276.

Padgett, Martin Jr. "Instant Gratification." *Prevention's Guide—Weight Loss*, October 1999: 30–33.

Papp, Leslie. "Breast Cancer Researchers Tell Women: 'Exercise Four Hours a Week.'" *Toronto Star*, June 19, 1999, A2.

Podleski, Janet and Greta. "Go Crazy!" *Homemaker's*, November 1999: 56–66.

Ranieri, Cathy. "Avoid Germs at the Gym." *Canadian Living*, November 1999:95.

Rhodes, Maura. "America's top 6 fad diets." *Good Housekeeping*, Vol. 223, July 1, 1996:100(3).

Ritter, Bill, Hugh Downs, and Barbara Walters. "The Shape of Your Marriage." ABC 20/20, October 9, 1998.

Salvadore, Dr. Steve et al. "Studies: Obesity kills but you can fight back." CNN.com, October 26, 1999: Health.

Saris, W.H. "Fit, fat and fat free: the metabolic aspects of weight control." *International Journal of Obesity and Related Metabolic Disorders*, August 1998; 22 Suppl. 2: S15–21.

Shea, Sarah Bowen. "The thin plan." *Men's Health*, Vol. 13, September 1, 1998: 96(3).

Shick, S.M. et al. "Persons successful at long-term weight loss and maintenance continue to consume a low-energy, low-fat diet." *Journal of the American Dietic Association*, April 1998; 98(4): 408–13.

Smith, Kerri. "Kerri's Story: UFOs of exercising." *Denver Post Online*, http://www.denverpost.com/life/kerri/kerri.htm, June 24, 1999.

Smith, Sally E. "The Great Diet Deception." *USA Today Magazine*, Vol. 123, January 1, 1995.

Snyderman, Nancy. "Eat Less, Exercise More, Eat Less, Exercise More..." *Good Housekeeping*, October 1999: 74.

Somer, Elizabeth. "Losing It." *Shape*, October 1999: 93–96.

Spilner, Maggie. "Break the weight-loss barrier." *Prevention*, Vol. 47, March 1, 1995: 82(8).

Stacey, Michelle. "Who isn't on a diet? In search of sensible eating." *Town & Country Monthly*, Vol. 150, June 1, 1996: 144(3).

Stanten, Michele. "71 weight loss tips that really work." *Prevention*, Vol. 50, March 1, 1998: 112(11).

Stanten, Michele. "PMS-induced bingeing." http://www.prevention.com, September 23, 1998.

Stedman, Nancy. "'It worked for me!' 25 slimming secrets from 5 weight loss winners." *Prevention*, Vol. 50, September 1, 1998: 124(10).

Stein, Joel. "Health: The Low-Carb Diet Craze Fad diets come and go, but this one is exploding. Can you really lose weight by feasting on beef, eggs and bacon? And should you?" *Time*, November 1, 1999: 72+.

Thomas, David. "Dangerous Dieting: Weight-loss fads can be hazardous to the health." *Maclean's*, February 10, 1997:54.

Tuomisto, T. et al. "Psychological and physiological characteristics of sweet food 'addiction'." *International Journal of Eating Disorders*, March 1999; 25(2): 169–75.

Wade, Nicholas. "Eating less is key to a longer life." *The Globe and Mail*, September 27, 1999, A19.

Wang, Julia. "Got a Few Minutes? We'll give You a Firmer Body." *Good Housekeeping*, October 1999; 42–44.

Wickens, Barbara. "Extreme Acts: Drastic shortcuts to slimness carry their own risks." *Maclean's*, January 11, 1999: 60.

Winick, Myron, MD. "Presentation Summaries: Research Update on Women, Weight & Dieting." Weight Watchers International, Inc., August 11, 1999.

Yeager, Selene. "Lose it by Liking Yourself." *Prevention's Guide—Weight Loss*. October 1999: 50–57.

Young Hwang, Mi. "Maintaining a Healthy Weight." *Journal of the American Medical Association*, Vol. 281, No. 3: 120.

Appendix F
Low-Fat Recipes by Pamela Steel

Blueberry Spelt Pancakes

Serves 4

Yes, you can still eat pancakes. We are splitting 1 egg between 4 people, which is completely acceptable. Using apple sauce adds sweetness without sugar and moisture without fat so, we only need to add 1/2 tablespoon (7 mL) of oil. Olive oil is not really the taste you want with your pancakes, so use canola oil instead. Pamela always uses organic spelt flour when baking at home to add variety to the grains in her family's diet, but regular all-purpose flour will work just as well.

> 1 cup (250 mL) spelt or all purpose flour
>
> 1/4 teaspoon (1 mL) baking soda
>
> 1/4 teaspoon (1 mL) baking powder
>
> Pinch salt
>
> 1 egg, beaten
>
> 1/2 cup (125 mL) nonfat milk
>
> 3 tablespoons (40 mL) applesauce
>
> 1/2 tablespoon (7 mL) canola oil
>
> 1/2 cup (125 mL) blueberries, fresh or frozen and thawed
>
> **Garnish:** Applesauce and blueberry yogurt make great toppings for pancakes and don't carry the calories of syrup.

1. In a large bowl, combine the flour, baking soda, baking powder, and salt. Make a well and add the egg, milk, applesauce, and oil. Stir together until smooth. Let rest, covered, for 30 minutes.

2. Heat a nonstick griddle or skillet over medium heat and spray with canola oil. If you don't have a separate sprayer for canola oil, brush the thinnest coat of oil possible onto the surface of the griddle. Pour 1 tablespoon (15 mL) of batter onto the hot griddle for each pancake. When the bottom has just set, drop blueberries into batter. When batter begins to bubble, turn the pancake and brown on the other side. Serve hot.

Nutrition:

Calories: 174.5

Protein: 5.7 g

Carbohydrates: 30.4 g

Fibre: .0.6 g

Total Fat: 3.2 g
  Sat: 0.5 g
  Mono: 1.5 g
  Poly: 0.8 g
  Cholesterol: 46 mg

Vitamin A: 149 RE

Vitamin B6: 0.06 mg

Vitamin B12: 0 mg

Vitamin C: 3 mg

Calcium: 70 mg

Iron: 1.7 mg

Potassium: 120 mg

Sodium: 166 mg

Zinc: 0.5 mg

French Canadian Soupe au Chou

Serves 4

The traditional version of this French Canadian classic calls for simmering a beef shank with onion and bay leaves for hours and then making the soup of its stock. If making a beef stock, let it sit in the refrigerator over night and then scrape off the hard, white fat layer before using in the soup. It's still a hearty soup with plenty of flavour when made with chicken stock and it won't eat up precious daily calories.

> 1 cup (250 mL) leeks, white only, chopped
>
> 1 tbsp (15 mL) olive oil
>
> 1 cup (250 mL) celery, diced
>
> 2 cups (500 mL) shredded cabbage
>
> 1/2 cup (125 mL) red wine
>
> 4 cups (1 L) low-fat, low-sodium beef or chicken stock
>
> 1 bay leaf
>
> Sea salt and fresh pepper
>
> **Garnish:** 3/4 cup (175 mL) carrots, grated

1. In a large, heavy nonstick saucepan combine the leeks and olive oil. Place over very low heat and cook gently for 5 minutes, then add the celery and cabbage. Cook for 5 to 10 minutes more, stirring frequently, until the onions and cabbage are completely softened.

2. Stir in the wine, the beef or chicken stock, and bay leaf, increase the heat to high. Stir until the mixture comes to the boil, then reduce the heat again and simmer for 30 minutes. Discard the bay leaf.

3. Pour into 4 warmed soup bowls and garnish with the grated carrot. Grind black pepper over each bowl and serve.

Nutrition:

Calories: 105.8

Protein: 12.3 g

Carbohydrates: 11.0 g

Fibre: 2.1 g

Total Fat: 3.6 g
    Sat: 0.5 g
    Mono: 2.5 g
    Poly: 0.4 g
    Cholesterol: 0 mg

Vitamin A: 11215 RE

Vitamin B6: 0.20 mg

Vitamin B12: 1 mg

Vitamin C: 21 mg

Calcium: 64 mg

Iron: 2.1 mg

Potassium: 482 mg

Sodium: 399.5 mg

Zinc: 0.7 mg

Roasted Acorn Squash and Garlic Soup

Serves 4

This soup is a winter-time favourite in Pamela's house. This is the time of year when nothing really grows in Canada so we look to our cold storage for ingredients like squash to cook with. Acorn squash is the small, dark green and orange squash that is shaped much like an acorn. Roasting the squash before puréeing it in this soup intensifies the flavours and brings out the natural sugar in the vegetable.

2 small acorn squash

2 bulbs garlic

Pinch sugar

1/4 teaspoon (1 mL) olive oil

3 1/2 cups (875 mL) low-fat, low-sodium chicken stock or replace some of the stock with infused milk

Garnish: 4 teaspoons (20 mL) low-fat yogurt

1. Preheat oven to 400°F (200°C). Cut squash in half and remove seeds. Chop tops off the garlic bulbs, revealing the tops of the cloves and creating a flat surface to season. Sprinkle with a pinch of sugar and drizzle olive oil on surface of garlic. Place squash and garlic on a tray in the oven for 45 minutes or until the squash is fork tender, the juices are seeping through, and the garlic is browned and bursting from its jacket.

2. In a medium saucepan, heat the stock and add infused milk, if using. Bring to the boiling point, then remove from heat.

3. When the squash is cooked, scrape the meat from the shell and place in a food processor. Carefully remove 4 cloves of garlic and reserve for garnish. Squeeze the remaining garlic into the food processor. Add half the stock and purée until smooth. Stir the puréed liquid into the remaining stock and warm through. Serve the soup in heated bowls.

Garnish: 1 teaspoon (5 mL) of yogurt with roasted garlic clove on top.

Nutrition:

Calories: 110.3

Protein: 12.3 g

Carbohydrates: 24.5 g

Fibre: 0.3 g

Total Fat: 0.5 g
　　Sat: 0.1 g
　　Mono: 0.2 g
　　Poly: 0.2 g
　　Cholesterol: 0 mg

Vitamin A: 560 RE

Vitamin B6: 0.47 mg

Vitamin B12: 0 mg

Vitamin C: 23 mg

Calcium: 104 mg

Iron: 2.3 mg

Potassium: 772 mg

Sodium: 232 mg

Zinc: 0.9 mg

Beet and Apple Cole Slaw

Serves 4 to 6

The brilliant colour of beets gives this salad a fantastic look. Serve it as a garnish with sandwiches or chicken, or as a brilliant side dish. Buy beets fresh with the leaves attached and use the leaves for a garnish.

   I small beet, grated

   I small red onion, thinly sliced

   2 small apples, peeled and grated

   1/4 cup (50 mL) nonfat yogurt

   I tablespoon (15 mL) Dijon mustard

   I tablespoon (15 mL) balsamic vinegar

   1/4 teaspoon (1 mL) salt

   4 beet leaves, optional

1. In a medium bowl combine the beet, red onion, and apple. Toss to mix evenly.

2. In a serving bowl, whisk together the yogurt, mustard, vinegar and salt.

3. Add the vegetables and toss together. Serve at once on washed beet greens, if you have them, or refrigerate for up to 48 hours. If the dressing separates, stir it together again.

Nutrition:

Calories: 53.0

Protein: 1.4 g

Carbohydrates: 13.1 g

Fibre: 2.3 g

Total Fat: 0.4 g
   Sat: 0.1 g
   Mono: 0.1 g
   Poly: 0.1 g
   Cholesterol: 0 mg

Vitamin A: 755 RE

Vitamin B6: 0.08 mg

Vitamin B12: 0 mg

Vitamin C: 8 mg

Calcium: 47 mg

Iron: 0.9 mg

Potassium: 249 mg

Sodium: 134 mg

Zinc: 0.3 mg

White Bean and Watercress Salad

Serves 4

This salad is an adaptation of a recipe from the Ontario White Bean Producers Web site. Their rendition weighed in at a whopping 13 grams of fat per serving. This is a perfect example of how a few easy tricks can help you adapt many recipes you find into low-fat versions. We have increased the ratio of greens to beans and substituted a dressing more suitable to our healthful tastes.

Dressing:

1/2 teaspoon (2 mL) salt

1 tablespoon (15 mL) balsamic vinegar

1 clove garlic, minced

2 tablespoon (25 mL) extra virgin olive oil

2 tablespoon (25 mL) chicken or vegetable stock

1 teaspoon (5 mL) Dijon mustard

Small pinch white pepper

1 cup white pea beans, precooked or canned, drained

2 cups (500 mL) watercress, large stems removed

1 stalk celery, sliced

1/2 small red onion, thinly sliced

1/2 red pepper, sliced

1 tablespoon (15 mL) fresh chives, chopped

1. In a medium serving bowl, dissolve the salt in the balsamic vinegar. Whisk together the remaining dressing ingredients set aside.

2. To prepare the salad, if cooking the beans, soak overnight in 4 cups (1 L) of water and then bring the same water to boil. Add beans and reduce to simmer and let simmer until soft, about 1 hour. Never salt beans until after they are cooked or they will stay hard. Rinse the watercress well and spin or pat dry.

Place the beans, watercress, celery, onion, and red pepper into the serving bowl and toss well to mix. Sprinkle the chopped chives over the top and serve.

Nutrition:

Calories: 244.3

Protein: 12.8 g

Carbohydrates: 33.7 g

Fibre: 8.8 g

Total Fat: 7.4 g
    Sat: 1.0 g
    Mono: 5.1 g
    Poly: 0.8 g
    Cholesterol: 0 mg

Vitamin A: 1307 RE

Vitamin B6: 0.24 mg

Vitamin B12: 0 mg

Vitamin C: 27 mg

Calcium: 152 mg

Iron: 5.6 mg

Potassium: 1045 mg

Sodium: 254 mg

Zinc: 2.0 mg

Smoked Mackerel with Spicy Garlic Foam

Serves 4

Smoked mackerel is another example of "good" fat. It is full of Omega-3 fatty acids, which current research suggests are beneficial in reducing the risk of breast cancer and may help to combat heart disease. The salad greens are served without dressing because the fish is flavourful enough as a topping on its own.

> 1 1/4 cup (300 mL) nonfat milk
>
> 1 clove garlic, sliced
>
> 1/4 teaspoon (1 mL) dried mustard
>
> 1/4 teaspoon (1 mL) dried chile pepper flakes
>
> 1 large handful mesclun (about 1 ounce/30 g)
>
> 4 ounces (120 g) smoked, peppered mackerel
>
> Salt

1. In a small pot, scald the milk with the garlic, mustard, and chile flakes. Use a spoon to strain out the garlic as you pour the hot milk into a stainless steel foamer. Pump until thick and voluminous, then set aside to firm up. Only the foam will be needed and the excess infused milk can be saved to make soup (see page 173). If you have a steam foamer, you will only need to use 1/2 cup (125 mL) of milk.

2. Divide the mesclun between four small plates and lightly salt. Cut the mackerel into strips and arrange on top of the greens.

3. Using a spoon, mound a dollop of foam over the mackerel and serve at once.

Nutrition:

Calories: 59.3

Protein: 8.5 g

Carbohydrates: 4.3 g

Fibre: 0.0 g

Total Fat: 0.8 g
 Sat: 0.2 g
 Mono: 0.3 g
 Poly: 0.1 g
 Cholesterol: 16 mg

Vitamin A: 365 RE

Vitamin B6: 0.17 mg

Vitamin B12: 5 mg

Vitamin C: 2 mg

Calcium: 106 mg

Iron: 0.6 mg

Potassium: 273 mg

Sodium: 321 mg

Zinc: 0.5 mg

Spaghetti with Roasted Red Pepper and Truffle Oil

Serves 4

In Italy, truffles are generously shaved onto pasta and the taste is so good, it's worth the flight. Flying to Italy is just a little less expensive than buying truffles here, but some of the flavour of Umbria can be brought to your pasta with truffle oil. The truffle is preserved in olive oil, which is a good fat, and the amount of flavour it packs is amazing. Yes, it's expensive, but a little goes a long way.

> 4 large red peppers
>
> 12 ounces (340 g) dried spaghetti
>
> 2 anchovies, minced
>
> 1 clove garlic, minced
>
> 1/2 teaspoon (2 mL) salt
>
> 1 tablespoon (15 mL) olive oil
>
> 1 tablespoon (15 mL) truffle oil
>
> 2 tablespoon (25 mL) parsley, chopped
>
> 1/4 teaspoon (1 mL) freshly ground black pepper

1. Preheat the oven to 450°F (230°C) and place the red peppers on a baking tray. Let roast for 25 minutes or until the skin is browned and blistering. Remove from the oven and place in a stainless steel bowl. Cover the bowl tightly with plastic wrap and let the peppers cool slightly. Peel the peppers and remove the seeds but retain the juice for the sauce. You may need to strain out some of the seeds.

2. Bring a large saucepan of salted water to the boil. Cook the spaghetti, according to package directions, until al dente.

3. Meanwhile, in a medium-sized bowl, combine the peppers with the pepper juice, the anchovies, the garlic, and salt and stir until the salt has dissolved. Stir in the olive oil and the truffle oil.

3. Drain the pasta well and add it to the bowl, tossing to combine. Check the seasonings, add pepper, and serve in warm bowls, sprinkled with the fresh parsley. Fresh Parmesan can be offered at the table for guests to shave onto the pasta as their daily fat allowance permits.

Nutrition:

Calories: 404.3

Protein: 12.4 g

Carbohydrates: 69.6 g

Fibre: 4.0 g

Total Fat: 8.4 g
  Sat: 1.2 g
  Mono: 5.2 g
  Poly: 1.2 g
  Cholesterol: 1 mg

Vitamin A: 1307 RE

Vitamin B6: 0.30 mg

Vitamin B12: 0 mg

Vitamin C: 143 mg

Calcium: 54 mg

Iron: 5.6 mg

Potassium: 352 mg

Sodium: 234 mg

Zinc: 1.3 mg

Grilled Corn on the Cob with Vegetable Medley

Serves 4

Nothing says "summer" like fresh sweet corn on the cob, grilled simply out of doors. The next time you fire up the barbecue, how about forgetting about the thick slabs of steaks and making a meal out of local vegetables? We've suggested a few, but your best bet is to go to your local farmers market, buy what looks nice and hurry it home for grilling. You're sure to come out with a feast you'll remember.

> 4 ears of corn in their husks
>
> I eggplant
>
> Olive or vegetable oil spray
>
> I teaspoon (5 mL) salt
>
> I teaspoon (5 mL) freshly ground black pepper
>
> I fennel bulb, top trimmed flush to the bulb
>
> 2 red peppers
>
> 4 portobello mushrooms
>
> 2 zucchini, sliced in rounds
>
> 8 artichoke hearts

I. Soak the ears of corn in their husks, in cold water, for 3 hours. Remove as much of the silk as will easily come away, before grilling. Any left in the husk will come away when you remove the husk. Grill on a hot grill for 2 to 3 minutes per side. The fresher the corn the better, and the less it needs to be grilled.

2. Cut the eggplant into I-inch (2.5-cm) rounds and sprinkle with salt. Place a weight over the rounds and let drain for I hour. Rinse and pat dry, then spray with oil and lightly season. Place on hot grill and cook for 5 to 7 minutes on each side.

3. Remove any bad spots from the fennel bulb, or if the outer layer is badly marked, remove it. Halve the fennel lengthwise, then cut each half into 2 or 3 pieces, depending on their size. Trim the core slightly on the diagonal, but do not remove or the wedges will fall apart. Spray with oil, season with salt and pepper and place on the hot grill for 5 to 8 minutes per side.

4. Place the red peppers on the grill whole, and turn when each side has turned dark and is blistering. Remove skin and seeds before serving.

5. Remove stems from mushrooms and reserve for stock. Brush clean tops, spray with oil and grill until soft and dark. The time will vary with the size and density of the mushrooms.

6. Lastly, spray zucchini and artichoke hearts with oil and lightly season. Place on hot grill and cook until grill marks are dark brown, 3 to 5 minutes per side.

Nutrition:

Calories: 195.4

Protein: 10.9 g

Carbohydrates: 43.2 g

Fibre: 14.9 g

Total Fat: 1.7 g
  Sat: 0.2 g
  Mono: 0.2 g
  Poly: 0.6 g
  Cholesterol: 0 mg

Vitamin A: 2893 RE

Vitamin B6: 0.50 mg

Vitamin B12: 0 mg

Vitamin C: 104 mg

Calcium: 121 mg

Iron: 4.0 mg

Potassium: 1461 mg

Sodium: 737 mg

Zinc: 11.7 mg

British Columbia–Style White Potatoes and Green Beans

Serves 4

This recipe was adapted from one that appeared on the B.C. Vegetable Marketing Commission's Web site. Their recipe weighed in at 18.6 grams of fat per serving and 316 calories, so we did a little doctoring of the ingredients. We cut the potatoes by half, increased the green beans, and substituted stock for most of the oil. Once again, we see how easy is it to adapt recipes to suit our low-fat lifestyle.

Dressing:

1 pound (500 g) B.C. or other white potatoes

2 cups (500 mL) fresh green beans

1/2 teaspoon (2 mL) salt

3 tbsp (50 mL) shallot vinegar

2 green onions, sliced

1 clove garlic, minced

1 yellow pepper, sliced

1/4 cup (50 mL) fresh chopped basil

3 tbsp (50 mL) chicken or vegetable stock

2 tbsp (25 mL) extra virgin olive oil

1/2 teaspoon (2 mL) freshly ground pepper

Garnish: Black pepper and basil.

1. In a large pot, cover potatoes with cold, salted water and bring to a boil. Reduce heat slightly and let simmer rapidly until soft, about 20 minutes. Drain, let cool and cut into bite-sized pieces.

2. Clean beans by snipping off the fibrous ends, cut into 2-inch (5-cm) lengths and then plunge them into salted, boiling water until the green colour becomes brilliant, about 3 to 5 minutes. Immediately refresh under cold water and drain. Cut each bean in half and set aside.

3. In a large serving bowl, make the dressing by dissolving the salt in the shallot vinegar.

Then whisk in remaining ingredients. Add the vegetables and toss until well mixed and coated with dressing.

Nutrition:

Calories: 180.9

Protein: 4.7 g

Carbohydrates: 27.7 g

Fibre: 5.0 g

Total Fat: 7.2 g
   Sat: 1.0 g
   Mono: 5.0 g
   Poly: 0.7 g
   Cholesterol: 0 mg

Vitamin A: 759 RE

Vitamin B6: 0.37 mg

Vitamin B12: 0 mg

Vitamin C: 109 mg

Calcium: 87 mg

Iron: 2.7 mg

Oven-Baked Fries

Serves 4

There are days when nothing but fries will do and when that day comes, this recipe can save you from trashing your commitment to healthy eating. It's still high in carbohydrates and calories, so keep portions modest.

> 2 large baking potatoes
>
> 1 egg white
>
> 2 teaspoon (5 mL) sugar
>
> 2 teaspoon (5 mL) chile powder
>
> 2 teaspoon (5 mL) paprika
>
> 2 teaspoon (5 mL) salt
>
> 2 tablespoon (15 mL) flour

1. Preheat the oven to 450°F (230°C). Wash potatoes and cut into strips 1 inch (2.5 cm) in diameter.

2. Mix together dry ingredients and spread on the bottom of a wide, flat baking dish.

3. Beat the egg in a large bowl until it begins to foam, then toss potatoes in egg. Pour potatoes into the baking dish and coat with the dry ingredients. Spread on a nonstick baking tray and bake for 30 to 35 minutes or until potatoes are browned.

Nutrition:

Calories: 78.2

Protein: 2.8 g

Carbohydrates: 16.6 g

Fibre: 1.6 g

Total Fat: 0.1 g
  Sat: 0.1 g
  Mono: 0.0 g
  Poly: 0.1 g
  Cholesterol: 0 mg

Vitamin A: 1134 RE

Vitamin B6: 0.14 mg

Vitamin B12: 0 mg

Vitamin C: 13 mg

Calcium: 11 mg

Iron: 1.1 mg

Potassium: 373 mg

Sodium: 571 mg

Zinc: 0.3 mg

Broccoli and Parmesan Stuffed P.E.I. Potatoes

Makes 4

Bud the Spud hails from the bright red mud of Prince Edward Island. Those wonderful, dirty, table potatoes have been a welcome staple in Canadian kitchens for as long as modern memory. Now, P.E.I. is also producing an equally good Idaho-style baking potato, ideal for this recipe. It is best to buy the potatoes from a bulk display so you can pick through them and choose not only the best, but also the smallest potatoes you can find. This will naturally reduce portion sizes.

> 4 small baking potatoes (about 4 ounces/120 g each)
>
> 1 cup (250 mL) broccoli florets
>
> 1/2 cup (125 mL) nonfat yogurt
>
> 1 tablespoon (15 mL) horseradish
>
> 2 tablespoons (25 mL) Parmesan

1. Preheat the oven to 375°F (190°C). Wash the potatoes and place directly on oven rack. Bake for 40 minutes or until soft to the touch.

2. Ten minutes before the potatoes are ready, steam the broccoli florets until they are brilliant green. If you don't have a steamer, they can be dropped into 4 cups (1 L) of rapidly boiling, salted water and cooked until their colour intensifies. Unfortunately, boiling destroys more vitamins and leeches out flavour.

3. Stir together yogurt and horseradish. When potatoes are finished baking, cut the skin away from one side. Scoop out the flesh and mix it with the Parmesan, then return it to the potato jacket. Arrange the broccoli over the potato with excess broccoli spilling over onto the plate. Serve with horseradish yogurt.

Nutrition:

Calories: 129.1

Protein: 6.2 g

Carbohydrates: 2.5 g

Fibre: 3.1 g

Total Fat: 1.1 g
  Sat: 0.6 g
  Mono: 0.2 g
  Poly: 0.1 g
  Cholesterol: 2 mg

Vitamin A: 573 RE

Vitamin B6: 0.38 mg

Vitamin B12: 0 mg

Vitamin C: 50 mg

Calcium: 117 mg

Iron: 1.2 mg

Potassium: 796 mg

Sodium: 86 mg

Zinc: 1.0 mg

Grain Patties with Roasted Garlic Yogurt

Serves 4

Eggs and cheese! Why not? When cooking low-fat, you will have much more success if you allow yourself to use these kinds of ingredients for binding, richness, and flavour. One egg and 1 tablespoon (15 mL) of Parmesan split between 4 people will contribute less than 2 grams of fat to your daily intake.

1/2 cup (75 mL) bulgur

1/2 cup (125 mL) couscous

1/4 cup (50 mL) fresh thyme, stemmed

1 egg

1/2 teaspoon (2 mL) salt

1 teaspoon (5 mL) dry mustard

2 tablespoons (25 mL) flour

1 tablespoon (15 mL) Parmesan

Olive oil spray

For Roasted Garlic Yogurt:

1/2 cup (125 mL) low-fat yogurt

2 bulbs garlic, roasted

1. In two separate bowls, steam the grains by combining the bulgur with 1 cup (250 mL) of boiling water, and the couscous with 1/2 cup (125 mL) boiling water. Cover the bowls tightly with plastic wrap and let the grains absorb the liquid and become tender, 20 minutes for the bulgur and 5 minutes for the couscous. Fluff the couscous with a fork to separate the grains.

2. Mix the egg with the thyme, salt, and dry mustard and stir into the grains. Dust the mixture with the flour and Parmesan and then stir until all is combined. Refrigerate for 2 hours. Form into 2-ounce (50-g) patties.

3. Heat a nonstick griddle or skillet over medium high heat and spray with olive oil. Brown patties on both sides, about 3 to 5 minutes per side.

4. To make yogurt sauce, roast garlic as directed, then purée with yogurt. Heat mixture in a stainless steel bowl over hot, not boiling water and salt to taste. Serve warm over grain patties.

Nutrition:

Calories: 174.2

Protein: 6.6 g

Carbohydrates: 26.3 g

Fibre: 4.4 g

Total Fat: 5.8 g
    Sat: 0.7 g
    Mono: 0.6 g
    Poly: 0.4 g
    Cholesterol: 46 mg

Vitamin A: 76 RE

Vitamin B6: 0.14 mg

Vitamin B12: 0 mg

Vitamin C: 0 mg

Calcium: 51 mg

Iron: 1.4 mg

Potassium: 156 mg

Sodium: 256 mg

Zinc: 1.0 mg

Bulgur in Savoy Cabbage Leaves

Serves 4

These rolls are a tasty low-fat take on traditional cabbage rolls. One of Pamela's favourite childhood family feasts was cabbage rolls and perogies from the local Polish delicatessen, served with gobs of fattening sour cream. These rolls offer the same satisfying heartiness. Take the time to make the roasted garlic yogurt and you won't even miss the sour cream.

> 4 leaves Savoy cabbage
>
> 3/4 cup (175 mL) bulgur
>
> 1 clove garlic, minced
>
> 1/4 teaspoon (1 mL) salt
>
> 1/4 teaspoon (1 mL) fresh ground black pepper
>
> Dash Worcestershire sauce
>
> 2 tablespoon (25 mL) chopped chives
>
> 1 cup (250 mL) canned plum tomatoes with juice
>
> 1 anchovy, rinsed and patted dry
>
> **Garnish:** A dollop of roasted garlic yogurt is ideal for these rolls

1. Preheat oven to 375°F (190°C). Bring 4 cups (1 L) of salted water to boil and plunge the cabbage leaves into the boiling water. Cook until they are soft and pliable, about 5 minutes, then remove from water and refresh under cold running water. Retain 2 1/4 cups (550 mL) of hot water for the bulgur.

2. Bring the water back to the boil and add the bulgur. Let it sit off the heat, covered tightly for 25 minutes or until all of the water is absorbed and the kernels are tender. Stir the garlic, salt, pepper, Worcestershire sauce, and chives into the bulgur.

3. Divide the mixture equally into 4 parts and spoon into the centre of the cabbage leaves. Roll the leaves as you would for cabbage rolls and place in a small baking dish. Cover with tomatoes and juice and cut the anchovy

into 4 thin strips. Place 1 strip over each cabbage roll. Place in the hot oven and bake for 30 minutes.

Nutrition:

Calories: 280

Protein: 19.5 g

Carbohydrates: 68.6 g

Fibre: 36.1 g

Total Fat: 3.2 g
    Sat: 0.5 g
    Mono: 0.5 g
    Poly: 1.6 g
    Cholesterol: 2 mg

Vitamin A: 6251 RE

Vitamin B6: 1.70 mg

Vitamin B12: 0 mg

Vitamin C: 181 mg

Calcium: 274 mg

Iron: 8.5 mg

Potassium: 2164 mg

Sodium: 1064 mg

Zinc: 5.0 mg

Smelts with Thyme and Pernod

Serves 4

Some of Pamela's fondest childhood memories are of fishing the smelt run at Point Pelee in southern Ontario. With her grandfather, she would go out into the water late at night and help reel in the big nets. Then came the gruesome job of cleaning hundreds of the tiny fish, but it was all worth it for the fishfry that followed. Of course, the fish were fried in tons of butter, but for this version we are frying them on a nonstick surface with just a spray of oil. Any loss of taste is more than made up for by finishing the fish with a splash of Pernod.

> 3 tablespoons (50 mL) flour
>
> 2 tablespoons (25 mL) fresh thyme, stemmed
>
> 1/4 teaspoon (1 mL) ground sea salt
>
> 1 egg white egg white
>
> 16 smelt, cleaned, head off
>
> Olive oil spray
>
> 3 tablespoons (50 mL) Pernod
>
> 2 lemons, cut in wedges

1. In a flat-bottomed, shallow bowl, combine the flour, thyme, salt, and pepper. In a second bowl, whisk the egg white until frothy. Dredge the fillets through the egg white and then lightly coat with the flour mixture.

2. Heat a nonstick skillet or griddle, preferably large enough to fry all the fish, over medium high heat and spray with olive oil. Quickly fry the smelts until browned on both sides, about 3 to 5 minutes. When the smelts are browned on both sides, add the Pernod and cook until absorbed. The Pernod may flame but it will extinguish itself in a second. If you are frying the fish in batches, wipe the griddle or pan clean between batches to remove any bits that may burn. Keep cooked smelts hot in a warm oven. Serve immediately, with wedges of fresh lemon.

Nutrition:

Calories: 382.7

Protein: 62.1 g

Carbohydrates: 10.6 g

Fibre: 0.0 g

Total Fat: 9.4 g
  Sat: 1.6 g
  Mono: 2.2 g
  Poly: 3.1 g
  Cholesterol: 238 mg

Vitamin A: 186 RE

Vitamin B6: 0.58 mg

Vitamin B12: 12 mg

Vitamin C: 42 mg

Calcium: 247 mg

Iron: 3.8 mg

Potassium: 1095 mg

Sodium: 338 mg

Zinc: 5.7 mg

Salmon and Mandarin Oranges in a Paper Bag

Serves 4

Paper-bag cookery is one of the prime choices for cooking fish. Here, fresh black bean sauce and shallots are paired together for a piquant surprise. The orange cuts the oiliness of the salmon in a charming fashion. This is an eye-opening dish, suitable for your gourmet friends.

> 4 16-inch (40-cm) square pieces parchment paper
>
> 4 1-inch (2.5-cm) salmon steaks
>
> 4 teaspoon (20 mL) black bean sauce
>
> 4 shallots, sliced
>
> 4 mandarin oranges, segmented
>
> **Garnish:** Serve on a bed of mesclun tossed in a shallot vinaigrette.

1. Preheat the oven to 450°F (230°C). Fold the paper squares in half and then reopen them to show the centre fold.

2. Place 1 steak in the centre of 1 side of each square. Rub in black bean sauce and sprinkle shallots over the surface of each steak. Cover with orange segments.

3. Fold the opposite, empty side of the paper over the contents and begin crimping and folding along 1 open side. Continue crimping all the way along to the other side of the folded edge, then fold the last corner underneath for added security. Repeat for the other 3 packets.

4. Place the packets on a large baking sheet and bake for 12 minutes, then serve the packets unopened, letting diners undo their own packets at the table.

Nutrition:

Calories: 257.9

Protein: 35.3 g

Carbohydrates: 12.6 g

Fibre: 1.7 g

Total Fat: 6.9 g
    Sat: 1.1 g
    Mono: 2.0 g
    Poly: 2.6 g
    Cholesterol: 88 mg

Vitamin A: 3641 RE

Vitamin B6: 0.47 mg

Vitamin B12: 5 mg

Vitamin C: 21 mg

Calcium: 43 mg

Iron: 1.8 mg

Potassium: 746 mg

Sodium: 304 mg

Zinc: 1.2 mg

Emmenthal Stuffed Chicken Breasts Braised in Tomato Sauce

Serves 4

Most Emmenthal cheeses weigh in at about 7 percent fat content, so although it is still a saturated fat, you can use it in moderation to make special dishes like this one. And it doesn't have the unpleasant texture of reduced-fat cheeses. Most chicken breasts weight at least 5 ounces (140 g), so trim them down to a 3 1/2-ounce (105-g) portion and reserve the trim for another meal.

> 1/4 teaspoon (1 mL) ground salt
>
> 1/4 teaspoon (1 mL) freshly ground black pepper
>
> 1 cup (250 mL) tomato sauce
>
> or
>
> 3/4 cup (175 mL) canned plum tomatoes in juice
>
> 1/4 cup (50 mL) red wine
>
> 1 clove garlic
>
> 1/4 cup (50 mL) chopped fresh basil

1. Preheat the oven to 375°F (190°C). When trimming the chicken, leave the thickest part of the breast and the tenderloin (the strip attached to the breast) for this dish. Place the chicken on a cutting surface with the side that would have had the skin on it facing down. Remove the tenderloin. Cut a pocket into the thickest part of the breast and place 1/2 ounce (15 g) of the cheese inside. Cover the opening up with the tenderloin and place the breast, tenderloin side down, in a baking dish. Season with salt and pepper.

2. Cover the chicken with store-bought or prepared tomato sauce, or combine the plum tomatoes with the red wine, garlic, and basil and pour this mixture over the chicken.

3. Braise, uncovered, for 20 minutes or until there is no pink left in the breast. Serve hot.

Nutrition:

Calories: 197.1

Protein: 28.0 g

Carbohydrates: 5.5 g

Fibre: 0.9 g

Total Fat: 5.6 g
  Sat: 3.0 g
  Mono: 1.4 g
  Poly: 0.5 g
  Cholesterol: 71 mg

Vitamin A: 813 IU

Vitamin B6: 0.66 mg

Vitamin B12: 1 mg

Vitamin C: 10 mg

Calcium: 162 mg

Iron: 1.4 mg

Potassium: 509 mg

Sodium: 593 mg

Zinc: 1.7 mg

Moroccan-Style Cornish Hens

Serves 4

Cornish hens are lovely to work with and their presentation is delightful. Here we have stuffed them with dates and apricots for a Moroccan-type treat. Removing the skin after cooking helps to keep these game hens moist.

2 Cornish hens

4 dried apricots

6 dates

2 tablespoon (30 mL) nonfat yogurt

Pinch dry mustard

1 clove garlic

1/4 teaspoon (1 mL) curry powder

1/4 teaspoon (1 mL) paprika

1. Preheat the oven to 400°F (200°C). Rinse the hens under cold, running water. Stuff the apricots and dates into the large cavity of the birds.

2. Combine the yogurt and spices and rub into the flesh of the bird. As much as possible, try to rub the seasonings under the skin so it is not all lost when you remove the skin. This is sometimes easier if you run a knife between the skin and the flesh at looser parts like the breast.

3. Roast the hens breast side down (to keep them juicy) on a roasting rack for 15 minutes. Reduce the oven heat to 325°F (165°C), turn the hens breast side up and roast for an additional 30 minutes or until firm with no trace of pink remaining at the thigh joint.

4. Let rest, loosely covered, on a platter for 10 minutes, then remove the skin, cut the hens in half and serve half per person with the fruits as garnish.

Nutrition:

Calories: 261.6

Protein: 24.2 g

Carbohydrates: 15.0 g

Fibre: 0.9 g

Total Fat: 11.6 g
  Sat: 3.2 g
  Mono: 4.5 g
  Poly: 2.5 g
  Cholesterol: 75 mg

Vitamin A: 1129 mg

Vitamin B6: 0.4 mg

Vitamin B12: 0 mg

Vitamin C: 1 mg

Calcium: 37 mg

Iron: 1.8 mg

Potassium: 419 mg

Sodium: 273 mg

Zinc: 1.8 mg

Lamb Loin with Shallot Jus

Serves 4

This is a very easy dish that uses the leaner loin cut of the lamb. The jus will be stronger if made with a lamb or beef stock, but chicken stock is often more convenient and works nicely. Pamela is fortunate enough to be able to buy organic lamb from local Ontario Mennonite farmers and the taste is too good to pass up, so she has devised several lower fat recipes like this one.

> 4 4-ounce (120-g) pieces of lamb loin, at room temperature
>
> Pinch salt
>
> Pinch freshly ground pepper
>
> Olive oil spray
>
> 2 tablespoons (25 mL) shallot vinegar
>
> 1/2 cup (125 mL) lamb, beef, or chicken stock
>
> 4 branches fresh rosemary
>
> **Garnish:** Place one branch of rosemary on each loin.

1. Preheat the oven to 400°F (200°C) and place a baking tray inside. Lamb loins tend to come in about 6-ounce (170-g) portions—too much for one, too little for two. Trim the loins to size and freeze the excess to make medallions of lamb at a later date.

2. Heat a nonstick skillet over high heat and spray with olive oil. Season loins with salt and pepper. When pan is very hot, brown loins on both sides, about 1 minute each side. Add vinegar and 2 tablespoons (25 mL) of the stock to the pan and let simmer for 30 seconds. Lift the loins out of the pan, letting all the liquid drain back into the jus and transfer the loins to the hot baking tray in the oven. Add the remaining stock to the jus and let reduce by half, then set aside.

3. Roast the lamb until it reaches desired doneness then remove from the oven—about 5 minutes for rare and 12 minutes for medium rare. Tent with foil and let rest for 5 minutes, then serve with jus drizzled on top.

Nutrition:

Calories: 74.1

Protein: 4.3 g

Carbohydrates: 0.8 g

Fibre: 0 g

Total Fat: 5.9 g
  Sat: 2.1 g
  Mono: 2.0 g
  Poly: 0.4 g
  Cholesterol: 16 mg

Vitamin A: 0 mg

Vitamin B6: 0.03 mg

Vitamin B12: 1 mg

Vitamin C: 0 mg

Calcium: 12 mg

Iron: 0.6 mg

Potassium: 90 mg

Sodium: 139 mg

Zinc: 0.8 mg

Berries in Warm Vanilla Foam

Serves 4

This dessert gives the luxurious mouth feel of whipped cream with a fraction of the fat and calories. Use fresh berries in season for their unbeatable taste. The pinch of chocolate on the top isn't enough to do any harm and it adds a scent of decadence to the dish.

> 2 cups (500 mL) mixed berries (any variety)
>
> 1 vanilla pod, split, or 1/2 teaspoon (2 mL) pure vanilla extract
>
> 1 1/2 cups (375 mL) nonfat milk
>
> 1 tablespoon (15 mL) honey
>
> 1/2 teaspoon (2 mL) chocolate shavings

1. Wash the berries and let them drain.

2. In a small saucepan, scrape the vanilla seeds from the pod, if using, and scald with the milk and honey by heating to just below the boiling point. Pour sweetened milk into a stainless steel foamer and add vanilla if using extract. Pump foamer until maximum volume is obtained, then put aside and the foam will firm up.

3. Portion berries into 4 cocktail glasses and top with a generous dollop of foam. Sprinkle a pinch of chocolate shavings over each serving. Serve with the foam still warm.

Nutrition:

Calories: 377.4

Protein: 15.0 g

Carbohydrates: 70.7 g

Fibre: 10.0 g

Total Fat: 6.6 g
    Sat: 3.3 g
    Mono: 1.9 g
    Poly: 0.6 g
    Cholesterol: 7 mg

Vitamin A: 938 RE

Vitamin B6: 0.29 mg

Vitamin B12: 1 mg

Vitamin C: 107 mg

Calcium: 495 mg

Iron: 1.6 mg

Potassium: 1046 mg

Sodium: 198 mg

Zinc: 2.3 mg

Strawberry and Rhubarb Crepes

Serves 4

Strawberry Rhubarb Pie is a great Canadian classic. The best ones are home baked but the pies that Pamela buys at her local Mennonite farmers market really are in a class by themselves. These crepes have the same spring-fresh filling of fresh strawberries and rhubarb but they are cooked down in unsweetened juice and served in very thin crepe shells.

For Shells:

1/3 cup (75 mL) all-purpose flour

Pinch baking powder

Pinch salt

1 tablespoon (15 mL) canola oil

2 tablespoons (25 mL) apple sauce

1/3 cup (75 mL) nonfat milk, room temperature

1 large egg, room temperature, beaten

Vegetable oil spray

3 stalks rhubarb, chopped

12 strawberries, sliced

1 cup (250 mL) unsweetened cranberry-apple juice

1 tablespoon (15 mL) Grand Marnier

Garnish: 1/4 teaspoon (1 mL) icing sugar

1. For crepe shells, sift together flour, baking powder, and salt. Make a well in flour and add the oil, apple sauce, milk, and egg. Whisk together, gently, until smooth. Let the batter rest for about 45 minutes. Place a nonstick or seasoned crepe pan over medium heat and spray with oil. Spoon 2 tablespoons (25 mL) of batter into pan and swirl to get an even coating. Let cook until the shell is lightly coloured on the bottom and set on the top—about 2 to 3 minutes. As each shell is removed from the pan, drop 2 even tablespoons (25 mL) of filling into centre and fold into an envelope shape. Note: If making the shells ahead of time, place a layer of waxed paper between each of them and store in the refrigerator until ready to use. This recipe will make 5 shells in case one tears or gets eaten.

2. While batter is resting, make filling by combining in a medium saucepan, the fruit and the juice. Heat over a medium high heat until the juice has reduced to a syrupy consistency, about 15 minutes. Add Grand Marnier and cook for an additional 2 minutes. Dust with icing sugar and serve warm.

Nutrition:

Calories: 299.5

Protein: 7.5 g

Carbohydrates: 53.8 g

Fibre: 13.4 g

Total Fat: 7.5 g
  Sat: 0.7 g
  Mono: 2.6 g
  Poly: 2.0 g
  Cholesterol: 46 mg

Vitamin A: 430 RE

Vitamin B6: 0.35 mg

Vitamin B12: 0 mg

Vitamin C: 274 mg

Calcium: 277 mg

Iron: 2.7 mg

Potassium: 1361 mg

Sodium: 77 mg

Zinc: 1.0 mg

Index